Table of Contents

Preface .... *v*

Section 1: **Exam Prep** 1

Section 2: **Self-Assessment Tests** 7

Section 3: **Practice Exams** 21

Section 4: **Answer Key** 111

Review Guide for the Certified Diabetes Educator® Exam

Fourth Edition

Contributors

Carol J. Homko, PhD, RN, CDE
Evan M. Sisson, PharmD, MHA, CDE
Janine Freeman, RD, LD, CDE, CDTP

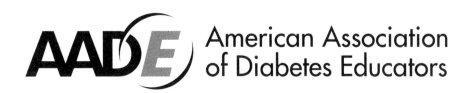

© 2017 American Association of Diabetes Educators, Chicago, Illinois.

First edition published 2007. Second edition published 2009. Second edition, revised published 2013. Third edition published 2015.

All rights reserved. No part of this publication may be reproduced electronically or mechanically, stored in a retrieval system, or transmitted in any form or by any means. The information contained in these files may not be copied to a diskette, mounted to a server, or otherwise distributed in any form without the express written permission of the American Association of Diabetes Educators. Printed and bound in the United States of America.

The views expressed in this publication are those of the authors and do not necessarily reflect the policies and/or official positions of the American Association of Diabetes Educators. Mention of product names in this publication does not constitute endorsement by the authors or by the American Association of Diabetes Educators. The American Association of Diabetes Educators and its officers, directors, employees, agents, and members assume no liability whatsoever for any personal or other injury, loss, or damage that may results from the application of the information contained herein.

10 9 8 7 6 5 4 3 2   18 19 20 21 22 23 24 25 26

Preface

Whether sitting for your first certified diabetes educator® (CDE®) exam or renewing your credential, the *Review Guide for the Certified Diabetes Educator® Exam* is your key study tool. The fourth edition is designed to help you assess your proficiency in the exam content areas.

The *Guide* begins by presenting strategies for preparing for and taking the exam. Next are three self-assessment tests based on the three content sections of the exam: Assessment of Diabetes and Prediabetes, Interventions for Diabetes and Prediabetes, and Disease Management. Complete these self-assessment tests to gauge the content areas for which you may require additional study.

The two, 200-multiple-choice-question exams replicate the experience of exam day. The questions are random and address topics from all three content areas.

An answer key for the self-assessments and the two practice exams provides the correct answer as well as an answer rationale for each of the more than 450 multiple-choice questions in the *Guide*.

Since eligibility requirements for the CDE examination change over time, the American Association of Diabetes Educators (AADE) strongly encourages you to check the website of the National Certification Board for Diabetes Educators (NCBDE, http://www.ncbde.org) for the most current eligibility requirements and the most current *Certification Handbook for Diabetes Educators*.

The NCBDE does not endorse, financially benefit from, or participate in the development of this exam review guide.

SECTION

1

Exam Prep
Strategies for Success

While studying is a critical part of getting good results on an exam, being adept at taking the test is also crucial. Fortunately, there are skills and techniques you can learn to help ensure test-taking success. These involve strategies for preparing for the exam, combating test anxiety, and learning how to assess each exam question.

First Things First: Know Yourself

In preparing for the exam, you will be most productive if you are aware of your study preferences, learning style, and daily functioning cycle. Having this knowledge of yourself will enable you to develop and engage in an effective study plan.

Start by identifying your best time of day. Are you a morning, afternoon, or evening person? Pinpoint your optimal time to devote to studying. When do you have the most time to devote to uninterrupted study: mornings, lunch hours, late evenings, weekdays or weekends?

Next, determine your learning preferences. Do you learn best working solo or in a group? Consider organizing a study group of other examinees if you learn well in a group setting. Be sure that you are studying in the environment that matches your own needs. This includes accommodating your physical space preference as well as understanding how much noise and distraction you can or cannot tolerate when you study.

What to Expect: About the Exam

The CDE® Examination is composed of 200 multiple-choice, objective questions. You will have a total testing time of four (4) hours. The examination is based on a content outline developed from a job analysis completed in 2013 that surveyed diabetes educators about the tasks they performed. Questions on the examination are linked directly to a task or tasks. As a result, each question is designed to test your knowledge necessary to perform the task or your ability to apply it to a job situation.

The NCBDE website includes a video on the computer-based testing procedures. Be sure to review it so you are familiar with what will occur on the day of your exam.

Changes and advances in medical treatment, diagnostic criteria, clinical guidelines, pharmaceuticals, and medical devices can occur at any point during a given year. Be sure to keep current as part of your study plan. The NCBDE recognizes that the dissemination of the information on advances may occur at different rates, depending on where you live. To address this disparity, the NCBDE developed the following policies:

♦ New medical advances, guidelines, or pharmaceuticals that impact diabetes self-management education and/or treatment of diabetes will be included in the Certification Examination for Diabetes Educators no sooner than one year after the information is released.

♦ New diagnostic criteria or specific guidelines that impact diabetes self-management education and/or treatment of diabetes that are released nationally and identified as effective immediately may be included in the examination at any time.

Getting Organized: Essential to Test Preparation

You will be better equipped to take the exam if you organize your preparation and sharpen your study skills:

♦ Allow ample time in advance of the test to study. Don't wait until the last minute.

♦ Review the *Certification Handbook for Diabetes Educators.*

♦ Draw up a time line for studying. Be realistic rather than overly ambitious.

♦ Develop a study plan based on the *Content Outline* in the *Handbook.* Use this as a guide for organizing your study time. Prioritize the content according to your strengths and weaknesses.

♦ Maintain consistency in following your study plan. However, be flexible when you need to be.

♦ Study in short and focused sessions. Be sure to take breaks.

Section 1: Exam Prep

Prepare Mentally, Physically, and Emotionally

Test preparation involves three components: mental, physical, and emotional preparedness.

To be mentally prepared, you need to learn and review all the material that will be covered. Review the *Certification Handbook for Diabetes Educators* so you are clear about the exam in terms of types of questions—the CDE® exam is multiple choice—time restrictions, and scoring (ie, how guessing and incorrect answers are scored).

In preparing physically to take the exam, be sure to follow healthful habits. This includes a nutritious diet, regular exercise, and adequate rest and sleep throughout the pre-test period. If you find it difficult to manage stress and have trouble winding down, practice yoga, muscle relaxation strategies, or rhythmic breathing.

Preparing emotionally for the test requires adopting a positive attitude, avoiding excessive worry, and bolstering your confidence. Because attitude often becomes a self-fulfilling prophecy, techniques such as positive imaging and positive self-talk can be vital during the period leading up to the exam. To promote a healthy frame of mind, create a mental image of yourself taking the test with confidence and performing very well. Envision the benefits that you will derive from obtaining the Certified Diabetes Educator® (CDE®) credential.

Exam Day: Focus on Assessing Each Test Item

When you sit down to take the exam, assess each test item. Start by determining the question type. Multiple-choice exam questions tend to fall into three categories:

1. Recall
2. Application
3. Analysis

Recall questions.   This type of question is asking you to remember facts, terminology, procedures, processes, definitions, and important principles. Identifying the current clinical guidelines for a diagnosis of diabetes and selecting the correct definition of the DAWN effect are examples of recall questions.

Application questions.   More complex than a recall question, an application question tends to provide a set of variables or a scenario. You are expected to demonstrate your ability to apply the information and suggest the next step in the process or the best way to resolve the problem. An example of an application question is a scenario that asks you to adjust the food intake for the patient described in the scenario.

Analysis questions.   These questions require more complex-level problem solving. A hypothetical situation is posed and you will need to synthesize the information and make judgments to determine which answer choice is the best or most appropriate response. An example of an analysis question is a scenario that ends with the question "What is the most likely reason for her elevated A1C level?"

3

Review Guide for the CDE® Exam

Based on the information provided in the rest of the scenario, you will need to analyze the situation and make a determination.

Next, consider the anatomy of the question. The *stem* of a test item identifies the specific question or intent, and may also contain background information. The *options* or *distractors* in a test item provide a list of possible answers.

In working a test item, keep these basic tips in mind:

♦ Find the key words or phrases in the stem of the question.

♦ Eliminate obvious wrong answers in the options.

♦ Narrow your choices and select the best option.

Following are five examples of the steps involved in assessing a test item:

♦ Example 1. Type of Question: Analysis

A 50-year-old man has recently developed diabetes. During the first education session, his wife frequently asks questions, often interrupting the educator's discussion with questions that are unrelated to the topic being taught. What is the educator's best option for managing this situation?

    A. Answer the questions and resume the planned course of instruction

    B. Discourage questions until the end of the class

    C. Allow several minutes for questions, then teach the topic of most concern to the husband and wife

    D. Remind the learners that there are important topics still to learn in a limited amount of time

Assess the stem: Find the important words or phrases: "recently developed diabetes," "interrupting," "unrelated," and "educator's best action."

Assess the options: Narrow the reasonable choices to two. Eliminate whatever does not make sense (options B and D). Think about what teaching/learning concepts apply to this case.

Best answer: Option C.

♦ Example 2. Type of Question: Analysis

The educator's best interpretation of the wife's behavior is that she

    A. is anxious about the anticipated lifestyle change.

    B. has a slow learning style.

    C. is dealing with denial and depression.

    D. has poor listening and comprehension skills.

Section 1: Exam Prep

Assess the stem: Find the important words or phrases: "best interpretation."

Assess the options: Narrow the reasonable choices to two. Eliminate whatever does not make sense. Options B, C, and D might be true, but not enough information is provided. (Experienced educators often try to "read between the lines" or overanalyze the stem.) Think about what psychosocial concepts apply to this case.

Best answer: Option A.

- ◆ Example 3. Type of Question: Application

  A patient reports that instead of taking her usual morning dose of insulin, she mistakenly took an extra 10 units of regular insulin. The educator would expect her blood glucose to

  A. decrease in 2 to 3 hours.

  B. increase in 6 to 8 hours.

  C. increase in 2 to 3 hours.

  D. decrease in 6 to 8 hours.

Assess the stem: Find the important words or phrases: "morning dose," "extra units of regular," and "expect blood glucose to."

Assess the options: Eliminate any answer that does not make sense, which includes any answer that says the blood glucose will increase (options B and C). Decide which of the remaining two answers is the best choice.

Best answer: Option A.

- ◆ Example 4. Type of Question: Recall

  Necrobiosis lipoidica diabeticorum typically occurs on the patient's

  A. shins.

  B. thighs.

  C. elbows.

  D. back.

Assess the stem: This is an example of an item in which the educator may have no idea what the question is. Analyze each word in the stem.

Assess the options: Look for similarities among the choices, because often options are written to test the ability to differentiate similarities. Shins and thighs have something in common because they are both on the leg. Therefore, cross off options C and D. Take your best guess with options A and B. In this case, it may be that the best you can do is narrow your choice to a 50-50 selection.

5

Review Guide for the CDE® Exam

SECTION 1: EXAM PREP

Best answer: Option A

♦ Example 5. Type of Question: Recall

A common symptom of cardiovascular autonomic neuropathy is

    A. a fixed heart rate.

    B. tachycardia with exercise.

    C. headaches.

    D. burning and numbness in feet.

Assess the stem: Note the important words or phrases: "cardiovascular," "autonomic," and "neuropathy." Think of related terms: heart/autonomic nervous system/complication.

Assess the options: Analyze each option. Option A: This could be bad if someone's pulse doesn't ever change (could be the answer as it is related to the heart and nerves responsible for rate). Option B: This is okay, since you *do* want the heart to beat faster with exercise; eliminate this option. Option C: Probably not related to the heart; eliminate this option. Option D: These are signs of peripheral neuropathy but *not* autonomic neuropathy; eliminate this option.

Best answer: Option A

Final Tips

Finally, keep these common exam pitfalls in mind as you take your exam:

♦ Read each question and all answer choices carefully. Be sure to catch important qualifiers, like "always," "never," "most," "least," and "typical," and the specific characteristics provided about the person in the question (eg, age, type of diabetes, comorbidities, medications).

♦ Avoid overthinking. Don't make assumptions that aren't supported by the question. Do not read more information into the question than is actually stated. Respond to the question as written.

♦ Don't become distracted because you think an entirely different answer choice that is not provided would be a better response to the question. One of the answer choices provided is the correct response.

♦ Don't look for patterns or sequences in the correct answer choices. For example, do not assume that "C" can't be the correct answer choice for three questions in a row. It can.

♦ Avoid wasting too much time on a few questions. You want to complete the entire exam.

SECTION

2

Self-Assessment Tests

Assessment of Diabetes and Prediabetes

1. A diabetes educator is consulted to provide discharge education for an 18-year-old patient diagnosed with type 1 diabetes. Upon entering the hospital room, the educator finds the patient quietly sobbing. The patient states that she is sad and anxious about her new diagnosis. Before the patient leaves for home today, which of the following should the educator review with the patient?

   A. Signs and symptoms of hypoglycemia and appropriate treatment

   B. Epidemiology of diabetes and the incidence of depression

   C. Incidence of birth defects associated with hyperglycemia

   D. Lifestyle modifications and carbohydrate counting

2. A 22-year-old patient with type 1 diabetes comes to the diabetes educator for additional education prior to starting on an insulin pump. During the visit, his cellular telephone rings, indicating a text message. Later, when trying to schedule a follow-up visit, the patient lays several other electronic devices on the counter while looking for his personal digital assistant (PDA). Which of the following is the best way to tailor future educational interventions with this patient?

   A. Schedule education sessions in the morning to avoid text message interruptions

   B. Offer online education for the patient to practice carbohydrate counting

   C. Politely ask the patient to leave his cell phone at home

   D. Enroll the patient in a group education class of patients with type 1 diabetes

7

Review Guide for the CDE® Exam

3. While covering the clinic for a sick colleague, a diabetes educator meets with a 56-year-old man who owns his own construction business. Despite the patient's apparent business success, his chart indicates that he is illiterate. Which of the following is TRUE about literacy?

    A. All patients will volunteer that they cannot read

    B. Most illiterate patients are poor, immigrants, or minorities

    C. Years of schooling is a good measure of literacy level

    D. Most adults who are illiterate successfully hide their literacy deficit

4. A 45-year-old truck driver who takes metformin and glyburide reports that he has tried to lose weight but nothing seems to work. Which of the following is the best follow-up question to address this patient's weight loss concerns?

    A. Do you carry glucose tablets with you to correct hypoglycemia?

    B. Did you know that weight gain can be a side effect of taking metformin?

    C. What types of foods do you eat when you are driving?

    D. How often do you check your blood glucose?

5. A 67-year-old man presents for evaluation of his glycemic control on glyburide therapy. He has not seen his primary care physician in more than a year. Which of the following diabetes-specific assessments should be performed today?

    A. Dilated eye exam

    B. Tuberculin skin test

    C. Lower extremity exam

    D. Gastric emptying test

6. A body mass index within the normal weight category is

    A. less than 18.5.

    B. 18.5–24.9.

    C. 25–29.9.

    D. greater than 30.

7. An intense fear of becoming fat even though underweight is characteristic of which of the following eating disorders?

    A. Anorexia nervosa

    B. Bulimia nervosa

    C. Binge-eating disorder

    D. Purging

Section 2: Self-Assessment Tests

8. Which of the following signs and symptoms suggests a diagnosis of hyperosmolar hyperglycemic state (HHS) versus diabetic ketoacidosis (DKA)?

   A. Hyperglycemia

   B. Dehydration

   C. Absence of ketosis

   D. Neurologic changes

9. Which of the following is an interfering factor that may affect the accuracy of A1C levels?

   A. Low doses of aspirin (81 mg)

   B. Sickle-cell hemoglobin

   C. High white blood cell count

   D. Oral contraceptives

10. GT was recently diagnosed with type 2 diabetes. Two weeks ago his primary care physician (PCP) placed him on a thiazolidinedione (TZD) despite strict adherence to a recommended diet and exercise prescription. The patient is discouraged because his self-monitored blood glucose levels remain elevated. Which of the following is the best plan for this patient?

    A. Review and intensify his exercise program

    B. Remind him that it can take up to 12 weeks to see an effect with a TZD

    C. Refer him back to the PCP for addition of another oral agent

    D. Further reduce calories in the patient's meal plan

11. A 51-year-old nurse with type 1 diabetes comes for education after her physician added pramlintide to her regimen. She reports improved blood glucose, but complains of occasional nausea about 30 minutes after injecting the pramlintide. Which of the following additional questions would be MOST helpful in evaluating the cause of her nausea?

    A. Do you take an aspirin every day?

    B. Was your dose of pramlintide recently increased?

    C. Do you get nauseated when you inject insulin?

    D. Do you inject the pramlintide into the muscle?

Review Guide for the CDE® Exam

12. A 53-year-old pastor taking metformin for 3 months presents to review his home glucose records. As requested, he has been testing his blood glucose twice daily for 2 weeks. Upon review, the diabetes educator notes that the 14-day average blood glucose of 130 mg/dL from his meter is much lower than the laboratory values from his lab work 2 weeks ago (A1C 11%, fasting plasma glucose 280 mg/dL, other routine lab work unremarkable). Which of the following is the best first course of action for the educator to resolve this discrepancy?

    A. Obtain a random non-fasting plasma glucose today

    B. Obtain a complete blood count (CBC) to check for anemia

    C. Assume the patient is falsifying his blood glucose record

    D. Have the patient demonstrate his self-monitoring of blood glucose (SMBG) technique

Read the following vignette to answer the next 2 questions.

A 72-year-old woman is referred to begin twice-daily insulin injections via vial and syringe. Additional known information

- Lives alone
- Limited income
- Polypharmacy
- Prescribed insulin: 70/30 premixed insulin, 17 units before breakfast, 14 units before supper

13. Since she will be taking insulin via vial and syringe, which physical capability is particularly important to assess?

    A. Dexterity and visual acuity

    B. Balance

    C. Hearing

    D. Visual acuity and hearing

14. What other potential barrier to effective insulin therapy warrants assessment?

    A. Diminished taste

    B. Financial concerns

    C. Altered pain perception

    D. Physical activity

15. A 45-year-old nurse has been newly diagnosed with type 2 diabetes and presents for education. What should the diabetes educator do first?

    A. Provide a detailed overview of the pathophysiology of type 2 diabetes

    B. Review a carbohydrate counting meal plan

    C. Assess the individual's interests, needs, and problems

    D. Discuss chronic complication risks

Interventions for Diabetes and Prediabetes

1. A middle-aged woman verbalizes understanding of meal planning concepts but consistently makes poor choices when dining out. Which of the following is the MOST appropriate approach for this patient?

   A. Suggest that the patient consult her doctor about social anxiety

   B. Use a menu and role-playing to enhance problem solving

   C. Advise the patient to avoid eating out as much as possible

   D. Discuss appropriate meal planning while dining out

2. A diabetes educator who provides service to 3 hospitals is designing an education program for school-aged children. Which of the following is the MOST appropriate teaching strategy for this population?

   A. An education sheet that automatically prints with the discharge instructions

   B. A prerecorded presentation with slides available on the hospital website

   C. A computer-based game about what impacts glycemic control

   D. A 45-minute live lecture provided monthly at each location

3. Which of the following is the MOST effective teaching method for self-monitoring of blood glucose?

   A. Lecture

   B. Print materials

   C. Demonstration

   D. Role-playing

4. Which of the following is the most appropriate treatment for hypoglycemia in a patient with type 2 diabetes treated with insulin or a sulfonylurea based on current ADA recommendations?

   A. Turkey (2 oz.) and cheese (1 oz.) sandwich

   B. 5 Saltines with 3 oz. cheese

   C. 5 oz. Greek yogurt

   D. 2–3 Tbs. raisins

5. Which of the following is the MOST appropriate recommendation for an individual with hypoglycemia unawareness?

   A. Avoid driving and always carry hypoglycemia treatment

   B. Check blood glucose before driving and always carry hypoglycemia treatment

   C. Consume carbohydrate every 4 hours while driving

   D. Check blood glucose every 30 minutes while driving

Review Guide for the CDE® Exam

6. A 34-year-old pregnant woman with suspected gestational diabetes presents for follow-up. She reports increased urinary frequency several times since her last visit. Which of the following is the best method to evaluate her current glycemic control?

   A. A1C

   B. Urinary ketones

   C. Fructosamine

   D. Microalbumin

7. According to the American Diabetes Association (ADA), an A1C less than 7.5% is the recommended target for children and adolescents

   A. less than 6 years of age.

   B. between the ages of 6 and 12 (children).

   C. between the ages of 13 and 18 (adolescents).

   D. across all age groups.

8. A 46-year-old female patient with newly diagnosed diabetes and hypertension complains that she does not want to start any medication. Her current blood pressure is 148/94 mm Hg. She is 5'3", weighs 158 lbs, and has a body mass index (BMI) of 28. Which of the following behavioral changes would have the greatest impact on her blood pressure?

   A. Lose 20 lbs through planned weight loss

   B. Restrict dietary sodium intake

   C. Exercise 20 minutes twice each week

   D. Restrict alcohol to fewer than 3 drinks per day

9. Alcohol consumption by individuals using insulin or insulin secretagogues can increase

   A. ketone production.

   B. gluconeogenesis.

   C. risk of hyperglycemia.

   D. risk of hypoglycemia.

10. At the conclusion of a general diabetes education group class, a 55-year-old man sitting in the back proudly announces that he plans to start training for the upcoming marathon. He reports being a runner in high school, but has not done any exercise since his popliteal bypass surgery 10 years ago. Which of the following is the MOST appropriate response to this announcement?

   A. Advise him to first obtain a graded exercise test with electrocardiogram

   B. Encourage the patient to walk for the first 20 minutes, then start running

   C. Encourage him to check his blood glucose after every mile of consistent walking

   D. Advise the patient that pain at night while at rest signifies improvement

Section 2: Self-Assessment Tests

11. Benefits of exercise include
    A. improved insulin sensitivity, increase in high-density lipoprotein, improved strength and physical work capacity.
    B. improved insulin sensitivity, increase in low-density lipoprotein, decreased fibrinolysis.
    C. improved strength and physical work capacity, decreased risk factors for coronary artery disease, decreased high-density lipoprotein.
    D. reduction in plasma cholesterol and triglycerides, decreased insulin sensitivity, decreased fibrinolysis.

12. A newly diagnosed 28-year-old patient comes to the diabetes educator for insulin injection training. Which of the following is MOST appropriately reserved for a follow-up visit?
    A. Proper insulin vial storage
    B. Insulin adjustment for sick days
    C. Preparation of the insulin dose
    D. Safe disposal of needles and syringes

13. An obese 50-year-old man with recently diagnosed type 2 diabetes and no other medical conditions inquires why his doctor started him on metformin instead of another agent. Which of the following is the MOST appropriate response to this query?
    A. Metformin was chosen, but a sulfonylurea could have been chosen because sulfonylureas do not cause weight gain or hypoglycemia
    B. Metformin was chosen because it is weight neutral and does not cause hypoglycemia
    C. Metformin was chosen, but a TZD could have been chosen as an inexpensive option that does not cause weight gain
    D. Metformin was chosen, but repaglinide could have been chosen since it doses only once a day and does not cause hypoglycemia

14. A 53-year-old male with a history of type 2 diabetes, hypercholesterolemia, coronary artery disease, hypertension, and erectile dysfunction presents for follow-up of his fasting laboratory results. The results showed

    - Total cholesterol 220 mg/dL
    - Triglycerides 128 mg/dL
    - LDL cholesterol 142 mg/dL
    - HDL cholesterol 32 mg/dL

    Which of the following lipid profile levels is currently at goal?
    A. Total cholesterol
    B. Triglycerides
    C. LDL cholesterol
    D. HDL cholesterol

Review Guide for the CDE® Exam

15. After his primary care appointment, a patient presents 2 new prescriptions for glargine insulin and lispro insulin to the diabetes educator. The patient has been taking NPH insulin and lispro insulin for several years and feels very comfortable with this combination. Which of the following is the MOST important counseling point for the patient today?

    A. Glargine insulin is stable at an acidic pH and must not be mixed with any other insulin in the same syringe

    B. Glargine insulin is 5 times more concentrated than NPH insulin, so only doses less than 0.2 mL should be injected

    C. Glargine insulin and lispro insulin are both clear, so care must be taken when mixing the two in a syringe

    D. Glargine insulin crystallizes when injected subcutaneously, and no other insulin should be injected within 60 minutes

16. The act of examining processes and outcomes to determine whether the desired goals and objectives were achieved is called

    A. evaluation.

    B. continuous quality improvement.

    C. outcomes monitoring.

    D. outcomes measurement.

17. Central obesity increases insulin resistance by which of the following mechanisms?

    A. Increased free fatty acid mobilization

    B. Decreased lipolysis in visceral fat cells

    C. Decreased glucose output from the liver

    D. Inactivation of insulin in the pancreas

18. FM's insulin-to-carbohydrate ratio is 1:12. His correction factor is 1 unit of rapid-acting insulin per 50 mg/dL of glucose. His target is 100 mg/dL, his prebreakfast blood glucose is 205 mg/dL, and he calculates the carbohydrate in his breakfast to be 50 g. Which of the following is the MOST appropriate aspart insulin dose for this patient?

    A. 3 units

    B. 4 units

    C. 5 units

    D. 6 units

Section 2: Self-Assessment Tests

19. A 37-year-old female aerobics instructor with type 1 diabetes presents to the diabetes educator for follow-up. She reports that she exercises 3 to 4 hours daily and that her weight has steadily dropped over the past few months. At this visit she weighs 110 lbs, her body mass index is 17, and her fasting plasma glucose is 290 mg/dL. Which of the following is the MOST important consideration when evaluating her glycemic control?

    A. The patient should be advised to eat a snack before exercising

    B. Her elevated glucose is likely reflective of the honeymoon phenomenon

    C. A psychiatrist should be consulted to evaluate the patient for an eating disorder

    D. She should consider increasing her basal insulin on exercise days

20. A woman with poorly controlled diabetes and peripheral neuropathy complains of a painful corn on her right foot. What is the MOST appropriate advice to give this patient?

    A. Advise her to consult with a pharmacist to select a corn remover

    B. Advise her to consult with a podiatrist

    C. Recommend that she purchase a sterile scalpel to cut away the dead skin

    D. Direct her to rub alcohol on her feet twice daily

21. A medical intern calls the inpatient pharmacist for a recommendation on starting insulin therapy for a patient who is 63 years old and weighs 220 lbs. The hospital protocol suggests starting basal insulin at 0.25 units/kg. Which of the following is the MOST appropriate starting dose of insulin for this patient?

    A. NPH insulin 55 units at bedtime

    B. NPH insulin 25 units at bedtime

    C. Detemir insulin 55 units at bedtime

    D. Glulisine insulin 25 units at bedtime

22. In the postabsorptive state (4 to 15.9 hours after food consumption)

    A. insulin inhibits breakdown of glycogen and triglyceride reservoirs.

    B. plasma insulin levels decrease and glucagon levels begin to rise.

    C. lactate makes up half of the gluconeogenic substrate.

    D. the rate of glucose being used by the brain diminishes.

23. Which of the following should be performed at every diabetes visit?

    A. Weight

    B. Fasting lipid profile

    C. A1C

    D. Dilated eye exam

15

Review Guide for the CDE® Exam

24. A 57-year-old male with recently diagnosed type 2 diabetes has a history of previous stroke, coronary artery disease, blood pressure of 180/82 mm Hg, and smoking 2 packs per day for 15 years. What referral warrants consideration?

    A. Referral to a registered dietitian for a consistent carbohydrate meal plan

    B. Referral to a registered dietitian for weight reduction

    C. Referral to a smoking cessation program

    D. Referral to a nephrologist

Read the following vignette to answer the next 3 questions.

A 36-year-old white female with a 7-year history of type 2 diabetes and previous history of gestational diabetes presents for diabetes education. She states that she has felt poorly over the past few months and that she is ready to make changes. Additional information known about this patient:

- 50 units of glargine insulin at bedtime and 30 units of regular insulin taken before breakfast at 9:00 AM and before supper at 6:00 PM
- Has a 6-month-old meter that requires a small blood sample and allows for alternate site testing
- Checks blood glucose 2 times daily, with results averaging 150 mg/dL before supper
- Recent A1C 9.3%
- Complains of extreme hunger and shakiness around 2 PM, with occasional blood glucose levels less than 70 mg/dL
- Does not follow any meal plan, but has a basic understanding of the effect of carbohydrate on blood glucose and often reads food labels
- 35 pounds overweight

25. Which meal planning approach best suits this individual?

    A. 1,200-calorie exchange plan

    B. MyPlate

    C. Carbohydrate counting with individualized carbohydrate goals

    D. Low-glycemic-index diet

26. Which of the following is the best recommendation to meet this patient's glycemic goals?

    A. Continue current doses of glargine and regular insulin

    B. Continue with glargine insulin, discontinue regular insulin, and add glipizide

    C. Discontinue glargine insulin, continue regular insulin, and add pioglitazone

    D. Continue glargine insulin and change regular insulin to aspart insulin before each meal

Section 2: Self-Assessment Tests

27. What information should this patient bring to follow-up visits to evaluate progress toward diabetes self-management goals?

    A. Blood glucose records and medication list

    B. Blood glucose records, food records, and most recent laboratory tests

    C. Blood glucose, food, and activity records

    D. Blood glucose, food, and activity records plus a log of insulin doses

Read the following vignette to answer the next 2 questions.

   JL is a 28-year-old female with type 1 diabetes and diabetic gastroparesis. Recently she has not been able to run for exercise due to nausea, vomiting, bloating, and intestinal pain. Her A1C is 6.7% and she reports experiencing hypoglycemia about 3 times a week.

28. What hypoglycemia treatment should JL use?

    A. Juice

    B. Regular soda

    C. Glucose tablets

    D. Peanut butter crackers

29. What nutrition modifications can JL benefit from?

    A. Consuming 3 meals a day, at the same time each day

    B. Consuming foods with soft consistency and increasing fiber intake

    C. Small, frequent meals; reduced fat and fiber intake; consuming foods with soft consistency

    D. Reduced carbohydrate intake and increased fluids

30. Which of the following describes normal hormonal response and the acute effects of physical activity?

    A. Insulin levels increase to reduce free fatty acid (FFA) production

    B. Glucagon rises and hepatic glucose production is increased

    C. Both epinephrine and norepinephrine are reduced and free fatty acid (FFA) production is inhibited

    D. Growth hormone and cortisol are decreased and insulin-stimulated glucose uptake is enhanced

17

Review Guide for the CDE® Exam

Disease Management

1. A diabetes educator in a university student health clinic is contacted to review the food records and carbohydrate counting skills of a college student with type 1 diabetes. The student explains that she has classes from 8:00 AM to 5:00 PM every weekday and cannot miss them to meet the diabetes educator. Which of the following is the MOST appropriate action for this educator?

   A. Offer to use the university e-mail system for follow-up with the student

   B. Suggest that the student come to the clinic at 6:00 AM, before her classes begin

   C. Offer to meet the student outside one of her classes to pick up her food records

   D. Ask the student to meet at a local restaurant on Saturday evening

2. A diabetes educator is asked to train patients on proper use of blood glucose meters. The educator has one meter and lancet device in the office. Which of the following is the MOST appropriate method to train patients and control infection?

   A. Clean the lancet device and blood glucose meter with soap and water after each training session

   B. Go over proper use of the blood glucose meter by reviewing the package insert with the patient

   C. Advise the patient to purchase a blood glucose meter and return to the office for training

   D. Demonstrate proper use of the blood glucose meter by lancing the finger of the diabetes educator only

3. A diabetes education program advisory board requests addition of an outcome measure directly related to the program curriculum. Which of the following is the MOST appropriate outcome measure to satisfy this request?

   A. Amputation rate among participants

   B. Frequency of physical activity

   C. Change in blood pressure over 1 year

   D. Average A1C level over 6 months

4. As part of a program's ongoing quality improvement process, a diabetes educator noticed a decline in the number of patients referred to the program over the last 6 months. Which of the following is the MOST appropriate response to address this decline?

   A. Assume that the number of patients with diabetes has decreased, and do nothing

   B. Assign more resources to television and newspaper advertising

   C. Change the format of the program from group classes to individual sessions

   D. Survey referring providers on their satisfaction with the program

Section 2: Self-Assessment Tests

5. How does a diabetes educator determine which portions of a diabetes self-management education program's written curriculum content areas are covered with a program participant?

   A. All content areas must be covered

   B. Assess the needs of the individual receiving the education

   C. Focus on the areas where the educator has the most knowledge and skills to impart

   D. Base upon desired program outcomes

6. The empowerment approach to education

   A. assumes healthcare professionals are the experts.

   B. utilizes instructions that are directive and uniform over time.

   C. promotes active participation in one's own care.

   D. is based on behavioral capacity and expectations.

7. You are seeing MJ for diabetes education. He tells you that he becomes very frustrated and agitated when his meals are delayed or when he experiences unexpected schedule changes. Which of the following would be MOST beneficial to his patient?

   A. Nutrition counseling

   B. Coping skills training

   C. Self-management training

   D. Problem-solving skills

8. To bring change in policies that influence community resources and support for persons with diabetes, it is important for healthcare professionals to be involved in

   A. exchange networks.

   B. advocacy work with state legislators.

   C. continuous quality improvement.

   D. community interventions.

9. Outcomes monitoring is

   A. how outcomes are used for educational and clinical decision making.

   B. the process of consistently measuring specific indicators.

   C. the frequency and interval of measuring specific indicators.

   D. the result from multiple variables over an extended time.

Review Guide for the CDE® Exam

10. A chart audit reveals that emergency room visits decreased by fourfold following participation in a diabetes self-management education program. Which of the following best supports the hypothesis that program participation decreased emergency room visits?

   A. More than 70% of participants subscribed to the monthly diabetes newsletter

   B. Over 90% of participants were highly satisfied with the program

   C. All program participants received a medical alert bracelet

   D. Medication refill compliance improved by 60%

SECTION

3

Practice Exams

Exam 1

1. A community pharmacy wants to offer a fee-for-service diabetes patient education program to its customers. Which of the following is the MOST appropriate way to market this new program?

A. Place an ad in the regional newspaper

B. Place flyers in every prescription bag

C. Send out letters to local hospital administrators

D. Contact the top 3 insurance companies in the state

Read the following vignette to answer the next 5 questions.

VA is a 46-year-old obese (BMI 33.9; weight 264 lbs) male construction worker who returns for follow-up. In addition to his vigorous job, VA also plays competitive racquetball 3 to 5 times each week. His past medical history is significant for coronary artery disease, type 2 diabetes, bladder cancer, hypercholesterolemia, and hypertension. He presents without new complaints today. He currently takes metformin 1 g twice daily, amlodipine 10 mg every morning, rosuvastatin 20 mg at bedtime, and aspirin 81 mg every morning. Today his blood pressure was 118/74 mm Hg and his pulse was 68 bpm. Fasting laboratory values today are as follows:

- Fasting plasma glucose 94 mg/dL
- A1C 8.2%

Review Guide for the CDE® Exam

- Serum creatinine 1.1 mg/dL
- Blood urea nitrogen (BUN) 18 mg/dL
- Total cholesterol 202 mg/dL
- Triglyceride 186 mg/dL
- LDL cholesterol 136 mg/dL
- HDL cholesterol 38 mg/dL

2. The physician would like VA to achieve an A1C goal of less than 7%. Which of the following would be the MOST appropriate addition to this patient's regimen?

   A. Glipizide 20 mg twice daily

   B. Sitagliptin 100 mg

   C. Glargine 60 units at bedtime

   D. Pioglitazone 15 mg daily

3. The physician would also like to specifically address VA's dyslipidemia at this visit. Which of the following is the MOST appropriate change to this patient's regimen?

   A. Increase rosuvastatin to 40 mg at bedtime

   B. Add fish oil 3 g twice daily

   C. Switch rosuvastatin to fluvastatin 40 mg daily

   D. Add ezetimibe 10 mg daily

4. The physician is considering adding niacin to VA's regimen but is concerned about hyperglycemia. Which of the following responses is most appropriate for this patient?

   A. Niacin impairs glucose tolerance and is absolutely contraindicated in patients with diabetes

   B. Gemfibrozil is a better choice for patients on simvastatin with low HDL cholesterol

   C. Patients with diabetes can use niacin, but the dose should be limited to less than 1 g

   D. Sustained release niacin is the best choice for patients with diabetes and low HDL cholesterol

5. Following a review of blood glucose logs 3 months later, VA was found to have an A1C of 7.5%. Which of the following is the MOST appropriate change to his regimen?

   A. Stop metformin and switch to glargine insulin twice daily

   B. Continue metformin 1 g twice daily and add glargine insulin at bedtime

   C. Decrease metformin to 500 mg every morning and add glargine insulin at bedtime

   D. Make no changes; VA is at his glycemic goal

Section 3: Practice Exams

6. VA heard on the news that calcium channel blockers increase mortality in patients with diabetes, so he stopped taking amlodipine. What is the best treatment plan for VA's hypertension?

   A. Start clonidine 0.3 mg three times daily

   B. Start irbesartan 150 mg daily

   C. Start hydrochlorothiazide 100 mg daily

   D. His blood pressure is fine where it is, so stop all antihypertensives

7. A 35-year-old woman with type 1 diabetes presents to the clinic for follow-up of self-monitoring of blood glucose (SMBG). Her A1C is 12%, and during the interview she reports that she thinks her boyfriend is interested in a younger, thinner woman. Which of the following is the best follow-up question related to this patient's concerns?

   A. Do you think that your boyfriend might stay with you if you become blind?

   B. Are you afraid that insulin might cause you to gain weight?

   C. Do your parents know that your blood glucoses are poorly controlled?

   D. What time of day do you check your blood glucose?

8. Routine labs for a patient with a history of normal glucose tolerance revealed a fasting glucose level of 113 mg/dL. What does this result indicate?

   A. Normal blood glucose

   B. Impaired fasting glucose

   C. Diabetes

   D. Gestational diabetes

9. SQ presents for a routine visit. While performing a foot examination you note "dependent rubor" (swelling and redness) when his feet are in a dependent position and pallor on elevation. Which of the following is the most likely explanation for these findings?

   A. Diabetic neuropathy

   B. Peripheral arterial disease

   C. Varicose veins

   D. Charcot joint

Read the following vignette to answer the next 3 questions.

You are seeing MN, a 36-year-old woman, for medical nutrition therapy, including basic carbohydrate counting. She has a 5-year history of type 2 diabetes and currently weighs 280 lbs. Her total cholesterol is 224 mg/dL and her LDL cholesterol is 130 mg/dL. A previous lipid profile from nearly 1 year prior showed total cholesterol of 193 mg/dL and LDL cholesterol of 99 mg/dL. During your assessment she shares with you that she is anxious most of the time, but not about anything specific; she feels that this anxiety is causing her to overeat and not be able to lose weight.

Review Guide for the CDE® Exam

10. Which of the following initial learning objectives is most appropriate for MN during this nutrition session?

   A. Identify carbohydrate foods

   B. Record food intake for 1 month

   C. Drink noncaloric beverages instead of soda each day

   D. Eat 3 servings of carbohydrates at dinner each evening

11. MN wants to know what lifestyle changes she should make to reduce her total cholesterol and LDL cholesterol levels. Which of the following interventions has the best evidence to lower total and LDL cholesterol?

   A. A weight loss of 3–5% if overweight or obese

   B. Resistance exercise of 30 minutes twice a week

   C. Replacing foods high in saturated and trans fats with foods high in unsaturated fats

   D. Drinking 2 glasses of wine each day

12. Which of the following would be the most appropriate referral?

   A. Cardiologist

   B. Nephrologist

   C. Social worker

   D. Mental health professional

13. An individual newly diagnosed with type 2 diabetes presents for education. What should the educator do first?

   A. Provide a detailed overview of the pathophysiology of type 2 diabetes

   B. Assess the individual's interests, needs, and problems

   C. Discuss chronic complication risk

   D. Review a carbohydrate counting meal plan

14. Which of the following medications should NOT be used in pregnancy?

   A. Human insulin

   B. Metformin

   C. Methyldopa

   D. HMG-CoA reductase inhibitors

24

Section 3: Practice Exams

15. A patient tells you that he wants to verify the accuracy of his meter. You tell him that the testing (meter vs. laboratory determination)

    A. should be done in the fasting state.

    B. is valid as long as he performs the testing 1 hour or less apart.

    C. result will be ~15% higher than the laboratory value if his meter reports whole blood glucose level values.

    D. should be done simultaneously using a drop of blood from the venipuncture.

16. FN has type 1 diabetes. When is testing for ketones the most appropriate?

    A. Daily in the morning after an overnight fast

    B. Prior to a decrease in insulin dosage

    C. With consistently elevated blood glucose

    D. Prior to exercise

Read the following vignette to answer the next 3 questions.

You are seeing LJ, a 14-year-old boy diagnosed with type 1 diabetes 2 months ago, for follow-up education. He tells you he has difficulty sticking with his meal plan when he is with his friends because they pressure him to eat high-sugar snacks.

17. Which of the following is characteristic of middle adolescence (aged 13–15 years) development?

    A. Increasing separation from the family unit

    B. Acute awareness of body image

    C. Peer group allegiance develops

    D. Cognitive abilities and abstract morals develop

18. Which of the following teaching strategies might work best to help LJ deal with this peer pressure?

    A. Games

    B. Discussion

    C. Role-playing

    D. Lecture

19. LJ's insulin requirements have decreased and his doctor has told him he is in the honeymoon period. Which of the following indicates how long this period typically lasts?

    A. 3 to 12 months

    B. Over 1 year

    C. 6 weeks

    D. 1 week

Review Guide for the CDE® Exam

20. A 73-year-old man with type 2 diabetes presents to the clinic complaining that he cannot pay for his medications any longer. He reports that the insurance copayment for one of his prescriptions went up from $5 to $100. Which of the following additional questions would be MOST helpful in assessing this problem?

    A. Did you go to a different chain pharmacy?

    B. Did you recently change insurance?

    C. When was the last time you had any prescriptions filled?

    D. Did you ask for a 3-month supply?

21. A single mother with type 2 diabetes is treated with 3 oral agents plus a bedtime injection of glargine. She presents to the clinic appearing disheveled. Her blood glucose log reveals widely fluctuating blood glucose values from day to day. She states that her days are filled with transporting her 3 children from one activity to another and that she does not have time for herself. Which of the following is the best way to address her fluctuating glucose values?

    A. Increase the bedtime insulin and monitor blood glucoses frequently

    B. Simplify her diabetes treatment plan to avoid missed doses

    C. Switch from oral agents and insulin injections to insulin pump therapy

    D. Ask the patient to keep a 3-month food plan diary

22. According to the National Standards for Diabetes Self-Management Education and Support, the instructional team for a diabetes self-management education program MUST include which of the following?

    A. Physician and a registered nurse

    B. Registered nurse and a social worker

    C. Registered dietitian and an exercise physiologist

    D. Registered nurse, a registered dietitian, or a registered pharmacist

23. An 86-year-old woman presents for an initial diabetes education evaluation. She lives in an assisted living environment and is unaccompanied today. She reports taking 15 medicines each day but does not know their names or their indications. Which of the following is the best source for additional medication history information?

    A. Contact the local pharmacy that fills her prescriptions

    B. Call the podiatrist that she visits each month

    C. Contact her daughter at work

    D. Have the patient identify drug pictures in the Physicians' Desk Reference® (PDR®)

Section 3: Practice Exams

24. A 45-year-old Hispanic man with type 2 diabetes for 10 years refuses to start insulin after failing oral agents. Which of the following is the MOST appropriate response for the educator?

    A. Educate the patient on the increased risk of microvascular complications

    B. Ask the patient why he does not want to start insulin

    C. Reassure the patient that insulin injections won't hurt

    D. Ask the patient if he has any family members with diabetes complications

25. A spotless blood glucose log from the past 2 months reveals twice-daily checks, with all results neatly written in blue ink and falling between 80 mg/dL and 125 mg/dL. An A1C drawn the week prior was 9.8%. Which of the following best summarizes the findings?

    A. The results correlate as expected

    B. The A1C is lower than expected

    C. The blood glucose values are not accurate

    D. The A1C was not fasting

26. Sad mood, lack of interest or pleasure, unintentional weight or appetite changes, fatigue, and worsening blood glucose control indicate the need for further evaluation of which of the following?

    A. An eating disorder

    B. Depression

    C. An anxiety disorder

    D. Anger management

Read the following vignette to answer the next 3 questions.

> JT is referred to the diabetes educator for education on self-monitoring of blood glucose. She sits down at the appointment with her arms crossed and states, "My doctor wants me to check my blood glucose more often, but I don't see the need for it. When I check twice a month it's always around 200 mg/dL and I feel fine." Additional known information:
>
> - 52-year-old married woman with 2 teenagers and her aging mother at home
> - Type 2 diabetes for 3 years
> - Owns a working blood glucose monitor
> - Recent A1C 7.6%

27. What should the diabetes educator do first?

    A. Reprimand JT for not checking more often

    B. Establish and maintain rapport with JT

    C. Remind JT of the complications that can result from uncontrolled blood glucose

    D. Reassure JT that checking twice a month is adequate

Review Guide for the CDE® Exam

28. In what stage of change is the patient regarding her blood glucose monitoring?

    A. Precontemplation

    B. Contemplation

    C. Preparation

    D. Action

29. Which AADE7 self-care behavior™ is most important for the educator to explore first?

    A. Healthy eating

    B. Monitoring

    C. Taking medication

    D. Being active (physical activity)

30. A 60-year-old man with cognitive deficits and dominant-handed weakness from a past cerebral vascular accident presents to learn how to inject insulin. Which of the following is the MOST appropriate method to assess insulin education successfulness?

    A. Ask the patient to describe the injection steps

    B. Have the patient write out the procedure

    C. Provide the patient with a pamphlet to take home

    D. Have the patient demonstrate an injection

31. Which of the following is the MOST effective way to determine the health literacy level of a person with diabetes who has been referred to you?

    A. Ask the patient how well he or she reads

    B. Obtain information about the individual's educational level

    C. Gauge the reading level based on the newspapers and magazines the individual reads

    D. Ask the patient to read an educational pamphlet on diabetes and explain its meaning

32. At the end of a nutrition counseling session, the diabetes educator asks the patient to pretend that the educator is a waitress and the patient is ordering a meal that would fit into her meal plan. This teaching format is called

    A. games.

    B. discussion.

    C. role-playing.

    D. demonstration.

28

Section 3: Practice Exams

33. Which of the following is the best method to prioritize diabetes learning objectives for the patient?

    A. Review of the medical record

    B. Recommendations of the referring physician

    C. Diabetes education curriculum

    D. Patient's identified interests or needs

34. A 24-year-old college student with type 1 diabetes presents to the pharmacist educator for insulin dose adjustment. She reports injecting the same amount of rapid-acting insulin with each meal and never makes any changes. Her recent A1C was 8.7%. Which of the following is the most appropriate approach for this patient?

    A. Advise the patient to search the Internet for information on meal planning

    B. Consult a registered dietitian to educate the patient about carbohydrate counting

    C. Telephone the patient's family to enlist their help and support

    D. Provide the patient with written materials to take home

Read the following vignette to answer the next 2 questions.

You are counseling PW, a 35-year-old man who was diagnosed with type 1 diabetes last week. He has just started on a basal/bolus insulin regimen that includes glargine (Lantus®) and lispro (Humalog®) insulins. His total daily dose of insulin is 55 units. He is motivated to intensify his blood glucose control but is concerned about gaining weight.

35. Which of the following is the MOST appropriate estimate of this patient's insulin sensitivity factor or correction bolus?

    A. 27

    B. 31

    C. 50

    D. 45

36. Which of the following referrals would be MOST appropriate for this patient?

    A. Clinical psychologist

    B. Registered dietitian

    C. Ophthalmologist

    D. Cardiologist

Review Guide for the CDE® Exam

37. Which of the following is the most appropriate sick-day management recommendation for patients with type 1 diabetes?

    A. Omit insulin when vomiting occurs

    B. Increase frequency of blood glucose monitoring

    C. Drink large amounts of carbohydrate-containing liquids

    D. Call healthcare professionals only if urine ketones are positive

38. "Record food intake, physical activity, and blood glucose results in a logbook 5 days a week for 6 weeks" is an example of a/an

    A. assessment.

    B. learning objective.

    C. behavioral objective.

    D. goal.

39. Specific, measurable, achievable, realistic, and time-bound (SMART) are characteristics of a well-developed

    A. learning objective.

    B. behavioral objective.

    C. action plan.

    D. evaluation.

40. TW is a 65-year-old man with newly diagnosed type 2 diabetes and low literacy skills. Which of the following teaching strategies would be most appropriate to implement?

    A. Use the same teaching approach as for all other individuals with diabetes

    B. State major learning points

    C. Use audiovisual teaching aids to cover all major points

    D. Include only TW in the education session to avoid distraction by family members/support persons

41. Which meal planning approach would best suit a 16-year-old with type 1 diabetes and normal body weight for height?

    A. 1,800-calorie meal pattern

    B. Carbohydrate counting

    C. 1,300-calorie meal pattern

    D. MyPyramid

Section 3: Practice Exams

42. Which of the following teaching strategies/formats best provides opportunity for on-demand, self-directed learning and problem solving?

    A. Discussion

    B. Print materials

    C. Role-playing

    D. Computers

Read the following vignette to answer the next 2 questions.

SP has just been diagnosed with gestational diabetes mellitus, and you are seeing her for diabetes education. Her current weight is 176 lbs and her prepregnancy BMI was 28 kg/m^2. Her fasting blood glucose is 135 mg/dL.

43. According to the Gestational Diabetes Mellitus Evidence Based Nutrition Practice Guidelines, women diagnosed with gestational diabetes should be referred to a registered dietitian for initial medical nutrition therapy

    A. only if the individual is overweight at diagnosis.

    B. within 48 hours of diagnosis.

    C. within 1 week of diagnosis.

    D. within 3 weeks of diagnosis.

44. Which of the following is the recommended total weight gain during pregnancy for this patient?

    A. 28 to 40 lbs.

    B. 25 to 35 lbs.

    C. 15 to 25 lbs.

    D. 15 lbs.

45. After 2 previous cancellations, a 67-year-old man with diabetes presents for blood glucose monitoring education. He states several times that he's only at the appointment to satisfy his doctor; however, he is fairly attentive and engaged until the blood glucose monitor is removed from the package. At this point, he begins to fidget and appears agitated. Based on this information, what would be the educator's best assessment of this man's behavior?

    A. Hypoglycemia

    B. Hyperglycemia

    C. Needle anxiety

    D. Short attention span

SECTION 3: PRACTICE EXAMS

31

Review Guide for the CDE® Exam

46. Which teaching method is the most effective form of active learning in a group education setting?

    A. Lecture

    B. Computer simulation

    C. Print materials

    D. Role-playing

47. A 19-year-old patient complains of unexplained weight loss and extreme hunger over the past month. Which of the following is the MOST useful information to confirm a diagnosis of diabetes?

    A. Patient reported polyuria

    B. A1C of 5.8%

    C. Fasting plasma glucose 106 mg/dL

    D. Random plasma blood glucose >200 mg/dL with polyuria

48. A 53-year-old man whose mother and brother have type 2 diabetes presents at a health screening. He asks, "How does the doctor know if I have diabetes?" What is the MOST appropriate response to this question?

    A. Your doctor may use an A1C test of 6.0% or greater to diagnose diabetes

    B. Type 2 diabetes must be diagnosed by HLA subtyping

    C. Your doctor may use 2 fasting blood glucose values over 126 mg/dL

    D. Type 1 diabetes can be diagnosed only if you are admitted for ketoacidosis

49. In the postabsorptive state (4 to 15.9 hours after food consumption)

    A. plasma insulin levels decrease and glucagon levels begin to rise.

    B. insulin inhibits breakdown of glycogen and triglyceride reservoirs.

    C. counter-regulatory hormone secretion is stimulated.

    D. excess glucose is stored in hepatic, muscle, adipose, and other tissue reservoirs.

50. LT has a recent A1C of 10.4% that rose from 7.2% six months ago. She recently stopped monitoring her blood glucose levels, complains of sleep disturbances, and says she has difficulty concentrating. Which of the following interventions is most appropriate for this patient?

    A. Screen her for depression

    B. Encourage her to enroll in a diabetes self-management program

    C. Reinforce the importance of blood glucose monitoring

    D. Work with her to set realistic self-care goals

Section 3: Practice Exams

Read the following vignette to answer the next 3 questions.

KB is a 59-year-old African American male with new-onset type 2 diabetes who is referred to you for instruction on self-monitoring of blood glucose (SMBG). He brings his meter to the session and tells you that he has read the instruction manual and watched the video. However, he expresses concern regarding his ability to test his blood glucose levels twice a day as recommended by his primary care physician.

51. Which teaching format is MOST appropriate for this patient?
    A. Lecture
    B. Online presentation
    C. Demonstration
    D. Print materials

52. According to the transtheoretical model, in what stage is KB?
    A. Contemplation
    B. Preparation
    C. Action
    D. Maintenance

53. Which of the following strategies would be MOST helpful in increasing KB's feelings of self-efficacy regarding self-monitoring of his blood glucose?
    A. Provide feedback to reinforce KB's successes
    B. Schedule a follow-up educational session
    C. Help KB identify the barriers to regular blood testing
    D. Recommend that KB join a support group

54. Which of the following islet cell antibodies is the best predictor of future type 1 diabetes?
    A. Heat shock protein 65
    B. Islet antigen A2 and A2 beta
    C. Glutamic acid decarboxylase
    D. Insulin autoantibodies

55. An overweight 52-year-old man presents complaining of polyuria, polydipsia, and fatigue. His fasting blood glucose is 326 mg/dL, and his urine is negative for ketones. Which of the following best describes the clinical presentation of this patient?
    A. Impaired fasting glucose
    B. Type 1 diabetes
    C. Type 2 diabetes
    D. Impaired glucose tolerance

33

Review Guide for the CDE® Exam

56. The Centers for Medicare and Medicaid Services (CMS) currently reimburses for

    A. 8 program hours of initial diabetes education and 1 hour in each subsequent year.

    B. 10 program hours of initial diabetes education and 2 hours in each subsequent year.

    C. 8 program hours of initial diabetes education and 2 hours in each subsequent year.

    D. 10 program hours of initial diabetes education and 4 hours in each subsequent year.

57. A woman at 27 weeks' gestation with previous normal plasma glucose levels undergoes a 100-g oral glucose tolerance test with the following results:

    - 92 mg/dL fasting
    - 196 mg/dL at 1 hour
    - 171 mg/dL at 2 hours
    - 152 mg/dL at 3 hours

    Which of the following diagnoses best describes the results of this test?

    A. Normal oral glucose tolerance test (OGTT)

    B. Inconclusive results

    C. Gestational diabetes

    D. Type 1 diabetes

58. A 14-year-old girl with type 1 diabetes presents accompanied by her mother. The girl sits quietly while her mother expresses concerns about her daughter's rising A1C. She adds that her daughter is tired all the time. "Instead of talking with her friends on the telephone, she just sleeps on the couch after school since not being selected for the school cheerleading squad 2 months ago." Which of the following best supports the diagnosis of adjustment disorder with depressed mood in this patient?

    A. Unintentional changes in weight or appetite

    B. Continuation of symptoms for more than 2 months

    C. Early morning awakening for at least 1 week

    D. Presence of manic symptoms (eg, excessive euphoria)

Read the following vignette to answer the next 3 questions.

GG is a 32-year-old Caucasian male with new-onset type 2 diabetes who is referred to you for nutrition counseling. GG has cognitive limitations but is able to live alone, and he prepares his own meals. A kind neighbor helps him with his medications and self-monitoring of blood glucose (SMBG).

Section 3: Practice Exams

59. During the initial nutrition assessment you should gather data on the patient's medical history, current medications, laboratory data, anthropometric measures, and
    A. a typical day's food intake and physical activity patterns.
    B. sick-day plan.
    C. insurance coverage.
    D. family support.

60. The assistance that GG's neighbor provides with his self-care regimen represents what form of support?
    A. Emotional
    B. Informational
    C. Instrumental
    D. Affirmational

61. Which meal planning approach would be most appropriate for GG?
    A. The plate method
    B. Carbohydrate counting
    C. Exchange list
    D. The DASH diet

62. A traveling salesman with type 2 diabetes for many years remains poorly controlled on 3 oral agents. He understands that high blood glucose is bad for him, but states that he does not want to start insulin. Which of the following is the MOST appropriate response to his proclamation?
    A. Do you think that you will lose your job if you start insulin?
    B. Are you afraid of giving yourself an insulin injection?
    C. What is it that concerns you most about starting insulin?
    D. Have you ever given yourself an injection with a syringe?

63. What should be the caregiver's role in diabetes management of a 14-year-old with type 1 diabetes?
    A. Drawing up insulin dose
    B. Providing physical and mental support
    C. Planning foods to be consumed at each meal/snack
    D. Perform blood glucose checks

Review Guide for the CDE® Exam

64. How often should individuals with diabetes have a dental checkup?

    A. Every 3 months

    B. Every 6 months

    C. Every 6 months and more often if periodontal disease is present

    D. Once a year

65. You are seeing AK for counseling. She has a 10-year history of type 1 diabetes and a 1% increase in her A1C since her last medical visit. She tells you that she became divorced 2 months ago and has been having difficulty functioning at work and following her self-management plan for several weeks now. Which of the following is the MOST likely diagnosis to accompany these symptoms?

    A. Major depressive disorder

    B. Adjustment disorder with depressed mood

    C. Dysthymic disorder

    D. Adjustment disorder with anxiety

66. The most commonly reported disordered eating behavior in individuals with type 2 diabetes is

    A. purging.

    B. bingeing.

    C. anorexia nervosa.

    D. insulin omission to facilitate weight loss.

67. A woman taking glipizide before breakfast and supper feels shaky, weak, and sweaty after walking for 30 minutes before lunch. She does not check her blood glucose routinely. She returns to the office, eats, and feels better after lunch. Which of the following is the MOST likely explanation for these symptoms?

    A. Hyperglycemia

    B. Hypoglycemia

    C. Overexertion

    D. Ketoacidosis

68. A patient on metformin monotherapy complains to his pharmacist about the high cost of the blood glucose test strips and asks why he needs to test his glucose at home. Which of the following is the most appropriate response?

    A. All patients with diabetes should test their blood glucose at least twice daily

    B. Self-monitored blood glucose is only useful for patients on insulin

    C. Self-monitored blood glucose lets patients see how food affects their glycemic control

    D. Urine testing is more appropriate for patients on oral agents for diabetes

Section 3: Practice Exams

69. Which of the following is the MOST frequent cause of inaccurate results from self-monitoring of blood glucose?

    A. Operator technique

    B. Improper calibration

    C. Expired or defective test strips

    D. Inadequate blood sample

70. MP was recently diagnosed with type 2 diabetes. Her doctor placed her on thiazolidinediones (TZDs) 1 month ago. MP is discouraged because, despite taking the TZDs as prescribed, her glucose levels remain elevated. Which of the following choices would be the best first step for a diabetes educator to do?

    A. Review her diet and exercise programs

    B. Remind her that it can take as long as 8 to 12 weeks of TZD use to see an effect

    C. Refer her back to her doctor for an addition of another oral agent

    D. Reduce the calories in her meal plan

71. You are counseling NL, who is on a basal/bolus insulin regimen. When evaluating her blood glucose records, which of the following would be MOST helpful to evaluate her basal insulin doses?

    A. Fasting blood glucose

    B. 1-hour postprandial glucose

    C. 2-hour postprandial glucose

    D. 4-hour postprandial glucose

72. A guitar player with type 1 diabetes does not test his blood glucose frequently because sore fingers interfere with his playing. Which of the following solutions is the best recommendation for this patient?

    A. Use a glucose sensor instead of capillary testing

    B. Avoid testing 12 hours before a concert

    C. Use urine test strips instead of a blood glucose meter

    D. Use a blood glucose meter with alternate site testing capabilities

73. A patient with previously good blood pressure readings has an office-based blood pressure reading of 147/96 mm Hg. What is the most appropriate plan of action?

    A. Blood pressure is in the acceptable range, so no action is necessary

    B. Recheck blood pressure at a 3-month follow-up appointment

    C. Confirm blood pressure on a separate day in the office or with home monitoring

    D. Initiate antihypertensive drug therapy today

Review Guide for the CDE® Exam

74. A 40-year-old man with type 2 diabetes for 3 years presents on his lunch break for diabetes education. Which of the following is MOST important for the diabetes educator to review with the patient at this initial visit?

    A. Economic impact of diabetes on the healthcare system

    B. Patient's family history of diabetes

    C. Patient expectations and personal education goals

    D. Pathophysiology of diabetes and its complications

75. A 12-year-old girl, accompanied by her mother, presents to the registered dietitian for meal planning. Which of the following is the most important consideration when developing her meal plan?

    A. Use the term "diet" instead of "meal plan" to emphasize weight loss urgency

    B. Schedule a separate session with the mother to review grocery selection

    C. Adjust the meal plan to meet energy requirements for growth and activity

    D. Suggest a plan that avoids intake of nutrient-dense foods

76. A 47-year-old woman with type 2 diabetes returns for a 3-month follow-up evaluation. She reports improved blood glucose and a 10-lb weight loss since her last visit. She states, "I feel great!" She continues to eat 3 meals daily and her exercise routine is unchanged. Which of the following additional questions would be MOST helpful in evaluating the cause of her weight loss?

    A. Did you stop taking your glipizide?

    B. Did you start taking a multivitamin?

    C. How much television do you watch each day?

    D. Have you recently made any changes in your beverage choices?

77. Which of the following tools is most useful to assess lifestyle activity?

    A. Blood glucose meter

    B. Pedometer

    C. Blood pressure cuff

    D. Holter monitor

78. An overweight 11-year-old Hispanic boy with type 2 diabetes presents to the registered dietitian for meal planning. His mother and father accompany him. Both are obese and have type 2 diabetes. Which of the following is the MOST appropriate advice for this patient?

    A. Avoid eating fast food

    B. Eliminate high-fat, calorie-dense foods

    C. Get involved in a soccer, basketball, or baseball league

    D. Aim for at least 60 minutes of moderate-intensity physical activity daily

Section 3: Practice Exams

79. The Nutrition Facts panel on a food package reveals 16 g of total carbohydrate per serving. How many carbohydrate choices (servings) do 2 servings of the food item contain?

    A. 1/2
    B. 1
    C. 2
    D. 3

80. In the Diabetes Prevention Program (DPP) study, which of the following interventions was most effective at preventing progression to diabetes?

    A. Troglitazone
    B. Lifestyle modification
    C. Omega-3 fatty acids
    D. Metformin

81. Olive oil and canola oil are sources of

    A. monounsaturated fat.
    B. polyunsaturated fat.
    C. saturated fat.
    D. trans fat.

82. When developing a diabetes self-management program, assessment of the target population should include assessment of educational needs, ethnic background, formal education level, reading ability, and

    A. knowledge about diabetes.
    B. attendance at medical appointments.
    C. social or family support.
    D. barriers to participation in education.

83. A 62-year-old woman with a history of type 2 diabetes and cardiovascular disease contacts the diabetes educator for advice on exercise. Her physician advised her to begin a resistance program following a recent diagnosis of osteopenia. Which of the following is the most appropriate exercise-related recommendation for this patient?

    A. Check her blood pressure and pulse frequently during exercise
    B. Focus on aerobic exercise to strengthen her bones
    C. Hold her breath while lifting to stimulate coronary perfusion
    D. Complete repetitions as quickly as possible

Review Guide for the CDE® Exam

84. An educator is hired to develop a new diabetes education program for an inner-city, hospital-based clinic. Which of the following is the MOST appropriate first step for this educator?

    A. Contact local drug industry representatives for education material

    B. Post flyers in the hospital waiting rooms announcing the education program

    C. Send out a memo to all hospital staff asking for referrals to the program

    D. Contact the hospital billing office to review patient demographic information

85. An obese 45-year-old patient expresses an interest in losing weight and asks for advice on exercise. Which of the following is the MOST appropriate exercise recommendation for this patient?

    A. Advise him that the real focus should be on meal planning, not exercise

    B. Encourage the patient to work up to walking 45 to 60 minutes for 5 to 7 days weekly

    C. Advise the patient that swimming is the best method to induce weight loss

    D. Recommend high-intensity exercise, such as running, for maximum weight loss

86. The Joint Position Statement on DSMES in Type 2 Diabetes indicates 4 critical times to assess, adjust, provide, and refer a patient for DSMES. Which of the following is NOT one of the 4 critical times?

    A. At diagnosis

    B. Six months following initial diagnosis

    C. Annual assessment

    D. When new complicating factors influence self-management

87. Which of the following should NOT be considered when assessing the physical capabilities and limitations of an individual with diabetes?

    A. Hearing

    B. Visual acuity

    C. Mobility

    D. Literacy

88. A patient with type 1 diabetes notes that her blood glucose prior to a 1-hour step aerobics class is 278 mg/dL. She has not taken any insulin since her last mealtime bolus. What is the most appropriate plan of action?

    A. Consume a 15 g carbohydrate snack to prevent hypoglycemia during the class

    B. Continue with the class because the exercise will lower the blood glucose

    C. Check for urine ketones and continue only if ketones are negative

    D. Skip the class and do not participate in vigorous exercise

Section 3: Practice Exams

89. A new billing clerk asks the diabetes educator for clarification about a Medicare patient. After an initial assessment, the educator indicates that the patient should be scheduled for an individual session instead of the usual group education class. According to Medicare regulations, which of the following is the MOST acceptable reason to schedule this patient for individual diabetes education?

    A. He prefers one-on-one education

    B. He is blind and reads Braille

    C. He takes insulin for diabetes

    D. He wears a hearing aid in one ear

90. Acarbose is added to glipizide to treat a patient with type 2 diabetes. Which of the following is the MOST appropriate recommendation to treat hypoglycemia in this patient?

    A. Orange juice

    B. Low-fat or skim milk

    C. Hard candy

    D. Regular soda

91. When collecting outcome data, a diabetes patient education program that bills Medicare must ensure that personal health information is always stored, analyzed, and reported in a manner that protects the identification of individuals as dictated by which of the following?

    A. Agency for Healthcare Research and Quality (AHRQ)

    B. American Diabetes Association (ADA)

    C. Health Insurance Portability and Accountability Act (HIPAA)

    D. Centers for Medicare and Medicaid Services (CMS)

92. A physician is considering adding metformin to a patient's regimen, but is unsure of how it improves glycemic control. Which of the following is the most appropriate description of the primary mechanism of action for metformin?

    A. Increased insulin sensitivity

    B. Inhibition of hepatic glucose release

    C. Delayed absorption of carbohydrates from the GI tract

    D. Enhanced insulin secretion from the islet cells of the pancreas

93. A postal worker who walks a route every day is newly diagnosed with type 2 diabetes. Which of the following drug classes is MOST likely to cause hypoglycemic symptoms while he is delivering the mail?

    A. Meglitinides

    B. Thiazolidinediones

    C. Biguanides

    D. DPP-IV inhibitors

Review Guide for the CDE® Exam

94. Which of the following is characteristic of quality improvement (QI) for an accredited diabetes education program?

    A. Systemic review of process and outcome data

    B. Conducted by management staff only

    C. Focuses on patient outcomes

    D. Quarterly reporting required by the National Standards for Diabetes Self-Management Education and Support (NSDSMES)

95. A 32-year-old woman with polycystic ovarian syndrome and newly diagnosed type 2 diabetes begins pioglitazone plus metformin. Which of the following should be included in her initial medication counseling?

    A. Use of contraception

    B. Hypoglycemia risk

    C. Risk for diabetic ketoacidosis

    D. Potential for disulfiram-like reaction

96. A patient on multiple daily injections reports frequent dawn phenomenon and between-meal hypoglycemia. Which of the following would be the most appropriate intervention for this patient?

    A. Institute carbohydrate counting

    B. Increase basal insulin dose

    C. Encourage more frequent blood glucose monitoring

    D. Initiate insulin pump therapy

97. Which of the following is consistent with serum glucose of 734 mg/dL, loss of 13% body weight, lethargy, mild confusion, and negative ketones?

    A. Hyperosmolar hyperglycemic state (HHS)

    B. Diabetic ketoacidosis (DKA)

    C. Insufficient insulin in type 1 diabetes

    D. Streptococcus infection

98. A middle school principal is concerned about the apparent rise in the number of obese children at her school. She has heard the reports in the media lately about the increasing incidence of type 2 diabetes in overweight children, so she contacts the local diabetes educator for recommendations. Which of the following is the MOST appropriate recommendation to prevent diabetes in the children?

    A. Organize a school assembly with presentations by a dialysis nurse and patient

    B. Encourage daily physical education and modify cafeteria food choices

    C. Write a letter to the parents of the children linking obesity and diabetes

    D. Offer a plasma glucose screening of parents at the school

42

Section 3: Practice Exams

99. Which of the following is characterized by the absence of warning signs of impending neuroglycopenia?

    A. Severe hypoglycemia

    B. Hypoglycemia unawareness

    C. Multifocal neuropathy

    D. Amyotrophy

100. In addition to increased serum ketones, diabetic ketoacidosis (DKA) is characterized by which of the following?

    A. Dehydration

    B. Decreased blood urea nitrogen (BUN) and serum creatinine

    C. Decreased serum osmolality

    D. Increased arterial pH

101. Which of the following oral agents is contraindicated in patients with New York Heart Association Class III or IV heart failure?

    A. Meglitinides

    B. Thiazolidinediones

    C. Alpha-glucosidase inhibitors

    D. Sulfonylureas

102. Which of the following is the MOST appropriate initial treatment goal for both diabetic ketoacidosis (DKA) and hyperglycemic hyperosmolar state (HHS)?

    A. Adequate insulin to restore glucose metabolism

    B. Correction of electrolyte deficits

    C. Rehydration

    D. Glucose replacement

103. Which is the MOST appropriate treatment for mild to moderate hypoglycemia?

    A. 12-oz can regular soda

    B. 4 oz juice

    C. 4 oz juice with 1 tablespoon sugar

    D. 1/2 peanut butter sandwich

Review Guide for the CDE® Exam

104. Which of the following best describes a patient with serum glucose of 359 mg/dL, arterial pH of 7.1, Kussmaul respirations, and electrolyte imbalance?

    A. New type 2 diabetes

    B. Hyperosmolar hyperglycemic state (HHS)

    C. Diabetic nephropathy

    D. Diabetic ketoacidosis (DKA)

105. A patient with type 1 diabetes telephones the diabetes educator stating that she has the flu. Her self-monitored blood glucose values are ranging 250–280 mg/dL, which is much higher than usual. She reports vomiting once, but now tolerates fluids well. Her husband just returned from the store with new urine ketone test strips. Which of the following is the MOST appropriate advice for this patient?

    A. Consume at least 8 oz of fluid per hour

    B. Make an urgent appointment with the endocrinologist

    C. Arrange for transportation to the local emergency department

    D. Contact primary care provider if urine is positive for small ketones

106. Including family members, friends, or significant others in the diabetes education session can help assess which of the following?

    A. Motivation

    B. Long-term outcomes

    C. Community support

    D. Social support

107. JC is a 63-year-old female with type 2 diabetes and an A1C of 7.8%. She has a sedentary job where she works at a computer all day. She would like to know how exercise can help lower her A1C. Which of the following is NOT a correct response?

    A. Daily exercise such as walking for 30 minutes can improve blood glucose

    B. Flexibility and balance exercises are recommended to improve glycemia

    C. Getting up from her chair and engaging in some type of light activity every 30 minutes when sitting for prolonged periods of time is advised for blood glucose benefits

    D. Not allowing more than 2 days to elapse between exercise sessions is recommended to enhance insulin action

Section 3: Practice Exams

108. A young nurse on a medical floor calls the diabetes educator to clarify why her patient with diabetic ketoacidosis is receiving potassium and insulin. Which of the following is the best rationale to provide the nurse?

    A. Suggest that low potassium levels usually resolve without supplementation

    B. Advise her that potassium should not be co-administered with insulin

    C. Insulin causes cells to take in potassium from the plasma

    D. Potassium is an essential cofactor for glucose metabolism

Read the following vignette to answer the next question.

A 32-year-old patient on insulin therapy is admitted with the following laboratory values:

- Serum glucose 750 mg/dL (reference 70–140 mg/dL)
- Serum osmolality 350 mOsm/kg (reference 275–295 mOsm/kg)
- Sodium bicarbonate 22 mEq/L (reference 22–26 mEq/L)
- Arterial pH 7.4 mmol/L (reference 7.36–7.44 mmol/L)
- Ketones SMALL (reference ABSENT)

109. Which of the following best supports the diagnosis of hyperosmolar hyperglycemic state (HHS) in this patient?

    A. Patient age

    B. Insulin therapy

    C. Serum osmolality

    D. Serum glucose

110. A 56-year-old patient with type 2 diabetes, uncontrolled hypertension, and chronic stable angina complains of inability to achieve an erection and asks about sildenafil (Viagra®). His current medications include glipizide 10 mg twice daily, lisinopril 20 mg once daily, and isosorbide dinitrate 10 mg three times daily. Which of the following is the MOST appropriate response to this patient?

    A. Suggest that the patient seek marriage counseling first

    B. Advise him that vardenafil is more effective, and offer to call his physician

    C. Suggest that the patient try yohimbine before starting prescription medications

    D. Advise him that sildenafil is contraindicated in patients taking nitrates

Review Guide for the CDE® Exam

111. A 45-year-old machine worker with severe peripheral neuropathy and an A1C of 9% is concerned about the possibility of amputation after his best friend with diabetes received a transmetatarsal amputation earlier this week. Which of the following is the MOST appropriate response to this patient's concerns?

    A. The risk of amputation is low in this patient due to his age

    B. Amputation risk is lowered by wearing shoes without laces

    C. Only patients with A1C values greater than 10% are at risk of amputation

    D. Daily foot inspections and proper nail care reduce amputation risk

112. A 53-year-old man newly diagnosed with type 2 diabetes and no other illness presents for initial diabetes education. Which of the following goals are MOST appropriate for this patient?

    A. A1C <6%, Microalbumin <100

    B. A1C <7%, Microalbumin <30

    C. A1C <8%, Microalbumin <300

    D. A1C <9%, Microalbumin <300

113. MS has been recently diagnosed with diabetes. She is having some difficulty managing her insulin regimen. She asks you if she will be able to go off insulin if she loses 25 lbs. This is an example of which stage of coping with a chronic disease?

    A. Depression and frustration

    B. Denial

    C. Bargaining

    D. Acceptance and adaptation

114. In addition to eating small, frequent meals, which of the following is the most appropriate recommendation for patients with gastroparesis?

    A. Reduce fat intake

    B. Reduce fluid intake

    C. Increase fiber intake

    D. Exercise before meals

115. When should individuals with type 2 diabetes have an initial dilated and comprehensive eye examination by an ophthalmologist or optometrist?

    A. Shortly after diagnosis with diabetes

    B. 6 months after diagnosis with diabetes

    C. 1 year after diagnosis with diabetes

    D. Within 5 years after diagnosis of diabetes

46

Section 3: Practice Exams

116. Which of the following statements about depression is TRUE?

    A. Individuals with diabetes have a 2- to 4-fold increased risk of depression

    B. Men with diabetes are twice as likely as women with diabetes to have depression

    C. Being older, married, and well educated are all significant risk factors for depression

    D. Cognitive behavioral therapy (CBT) has not been shown to be effective in treating individuals with diabetes and depression

117. According to the ADA Standards of Care, which dietary protein modification is recommended for individuals with diabetes and nondialysis-dependent chronic kidney disease?

    A. Less than 0.6 g/kg body weight/day

    B. 0.8 g/kg body weight/day

    C. More than 1.0 g/kg body weight/day

    D. Limit protein to 4 ounces per day

118. Based on The Seventh Report of the Joint National Committee on Prevention, Detection, Evaluation, and Treatment of High Blood Pressure (JNC 7) guidelines, a blood pressure of 150/95 mm Hg would be classified as which of the following?

    A. High-normal

    B. Prehypertension

    C. Stage 1 hypertension

    D. Stage 2 hypertension

119. Which of the following is the most prevalent oral complication of diabetes?

    A. Dental caries

    B. Periodontal disease

    C. Dental abscesses

    D. Burning mouth syndrome

120. Which of the following is the most common autoimmune disorder associated with type 1 diabetes?

    A. Celiac sprue

    B. Thyroid disorders

    C. Addison's disease

    D. Vitiligo

Review Guide for the CDE® Exam

121. Due to budget constraints, a diabetes educator is required to provide quarterly productivity reports. To facilitate generation of these reports, the educator decides to create a database. Which of the following are the MOST appropriate data elements to include in this database?

    A. Patient name and visit dates

    B. Behavioral change goals by patient

    C. Patient name and telephone number

    D. Baseline blood pressure and plasma glucose

122. An elderly patient complains that he has trouble reading the newspaper in the evening after dinner. He adds that his vision is fine throughout the day and becomes blurry only after he eats a large meal. Which of the following is the MOST likely explanation of his blurred vision?

    A. Nonproliferative diabetic retinopathy

    B. Macular degeneration

    C. Detachment of the retina

    D. Osmotic changes in the lens

123. A 22-year-old pregnant Caucasian woman asks if she should be tested for gestational diabetes mellitus (GDM). She denies any family history of diabetes and states that her obstetrician is very pleased with her weight gain during this first pregnancy. Her BMI is 22 kg/m². Based on current recommendations, which of the following represents the best response to this woman?

    A. Gestational diabetes is very rare and too many women are tested inappropriately

    B. All pregnant women should be screened for gestational diabetes regardless of the risk

    C. Screening for gestational diabetes is only recommended for women aged 25 or older

    D. Screening for gestational diabetes is only necessary for symptomatic women

124. Which guiding principle of motivational interviewing does the following statement demonstrate: "It sounds like getting routine physical activity is difficult for you due to long work hours, volunteer commitments, and young children to care for in the evenings. It's a common struggle. Where in your day might physical activity fit in, and what types do you enjoy?"

    A. Expressing empathy

    B. Developing discrepancies

    C. Rolling with resistance

    D. Supporting self-efficacy

**SECTION 3:
PRACTICE EXAMS**

48

Section 3: Practice Exams

125. A 26-year-old pregnant woman with preexisting type 1 diabetes presents for diabetes education. Which of the following is the MOST appropriate advice for this patient?

    A. Aerobic activity should be limited to less than 30 minutes per day

    B. Fasting blood glucose should remain between 60 and 100 mg/dL

    C. A1C values should remain 1% higher than the prepregnancy average

    D. Exercise should be initiated only if the blood glucose is greater than 200 mg/dL

126. Which of the following statements is TRUE regarding insulin requirements during pregnancy? The requirements

    A. generally decrease in the weeks before delivery.

    B. are highest immediately following organogenesis.

    C. are increased in late gestation.

    D. are lower in women with type 2 diabetes.

127. You are seeing KL, a 23-year-old pregnant African American woman who is at 8 weeks gestation and has a family history of type 2 diabetes. What is the most appropriate timing to screen her for gestational diabetes?

    A. At her first prenatal visit

    B. Upon presence of clinical symptoms (glycosuria)

    C. Between 24 and 28 weeks gestation

    D. At 20 weeks gestation

128. A 31-year-old married woman with type 2 diabetes and a recent A1C of 7.9% expresses a desire to become pregnant in the next year. Which is the most appropriate response from the diabetes educator?

    A. Recommend effective contraception until good metabolic control is achieved

    B. Encourage her physician to promptly initiate insulin therapy

    C. Maintain current A1C to prevent excessive hypoglycemia prior to conception

    D. Advise against pregnancy since she has diabetes

129. What is the term for verbal and nonverbal behaviors that people use to signal to another person that they are listening and the person should continue?

    A. Feedback

    B. Minimal encouragers

    C. Paraphrasing

    D. Clarification

Review Guide for the CDE® Exam

130. A 73-year-old male with good manual dexterity takes insulin via vial and 1 mL syringe. He states that his dose is "about 40 units at breakfast and about 52 units at dinner." When asked to demonstrate drawing up 52 units, the plunger is noted to be on 56 units. Which of the following is the best insulin delivery device recommendation for this patient?

    A. ½-mL syringe

    B. Insulin pump

    C. Insulin syringe magnifier

    D. Jet injector

131. The insulin needs of a teenage male with newly diagnosed type 1 diabetes are noted to be 1.0 unit per kilogram of body weight per day. Approximately 1 month after diagnosis, he contacts the diabetes educator complaining of frequent hypoglycemia. He denies changes in his insulin-to-carbohydrate ratio or physical activity. What is the most likely explanation for the hypoglycemia?

    A. Dawn phenomenon

    B. Somogyi effect

    C. Honeymoon period

    D. Spoiled insulin

132. The Diabetes Control and Complications Trial (DCCT) found that intensive glycemic control in patients with type 1 diabetes resulted in which of the following outcomes? Decreased risk of

    A. hypoglycemia but increased risk of hyperglycemia.

    B. retinopathy but increased risk of atherosclerosis.

    C. microvascular complications but increased risk of hypoglycemia.

    D. microvascular complications but only at A1C values <6%.

Read the following vignette to answer the next 2 questions.

    DF has been referred to you for preconception counseling and improved blood glucose control. She is recently married and is eager to have a child. She has a 10-year history of type 1 diabetes and was diagnosed with background retinopathy. She has several questions about many issues, but her major concern is the impact of pregnancy on her vision.

133. You establish which of the following as the primary learning objective?

    A. Discuss the impact of pregnancy on retinopathy progression

    B. Identify postprandial glucose targets

    C. List potential neonatal complications

    D. Discuss use of artificial sweeteners in pregnancy

Section 3: Practice Exams

134. Which of the following statements regarding retinopathy and pregnancy is TRUE?

    A. Rapid normalization of blood glucose values can halt progression of retinopathy

    B. Changes in retinopathy that occur during pregnancy tend to be permanent

    C. Pregnancy should be delayed in the presence of untreated proliferative retinopathy

    D. Hypertension does not alter the progression of retinopathy

135. Which of the following represents glucose targets during the preconception period?

    A. Premeal <95mg/dL; 2-hour postprandial <120 mg/dL

    B. Premeal <126 mg/dL; 2-hour postprandial <140mg/dL

    C. Premeal <140 mg/dL; 2-hour postprandial <189 mg/dL

    D. Premeal <155mg/dL; 2-hour postprandial <200mg/dL

136. A 26-year-old African American man with a strong family history of diabetes asks his local pharmacist if there is anything he can do to prevent diabetes. According to the Diabetes Prevention Program (DPP), what is the MOST effective intervention?

    A. Weight loss and at least 150 minutes of exercise weekly

    B. Acarbose 100 mg with the first bite of each meal

    C. Metformin 850 mg twice daily with food

    D. Rosiglitazone 2 mg twice daily

137. The Diabetes Prevention Program (DPP) demonstrated that lifestyle intervention reduced the risk of developing type 2 diabetes by what percent?

    A. 7%

    B. 15%

    C. 37%

    D. 58%

138. Based on the Diabetes Prevention Program (DPP), which of the following represents the amount of weight loss necessary to prevent type 2 diabetes?

    A. 1% to 2% initial body weight

    B. 3% to 4% initial body weight

    C. 5% to 7% initial body weight

    D. 8% to 9% initial body weight

Review Guide for the CDE® Exam

139. CC is a 62-year-old man with a 10-year history of type 2 diabetes and tobacco abuse, and he was recently diagnosed with cardiovascular disease. How should his lipids be managed?

    A. Low intensity statin and lifestyle therapy

    B. High intensity statin and lifestyle therapy

    C. Lifestyle therapy only

    D. Moderate intensity statin and lifestyle therapy

140. Which of the following statements is TRUE for all models of insulin pumps?

    A. Costs are approximately the same

    B. Have a plastic tube that connects the pump to the skin

    C. Deliver both basal and bolus insulin

    D. Will be appropriate for the needs of all users

141. Large daily doses of aspirin (approximately 4 g/day) can cause which of the following drug-disease interactions?

    A. Intrinsic hypoglycemic effect

    B. Decreased basal and inhibition of release of insulin

    C. Intrinsic glycemic effect

    D. Increased basal and stimulated release of insulin

142. RG has severe peripheral neuropathy, but expresses a desire to stay physically active. Which form of activity could NOT be safely recommended?

    A. Moderate walking

    B. Aerobics class

    C. Swimming

    D. Chair exercises

143. A patient states that he does not read much and left his glasses at home. He seems uninterested in written educational materials. Which of the following should the diabetes educator assess?

    A. Visual acuity

    B. Literacy level

    C. Language

    D. Mental acuity

SECTION 3: PRACTICE EXAMS

52

144. You are seeing BD for nutrition counseling. You perform an assessment and discover he is taking several dietary supplements, which include ginkgo biloba, bilberry, and milk thistle. Which of the following is the most appropriate response?

   A. Complementary therapies are generally safe because they are "natural."

   B. Dietary supplements have a low risk of side effects.

   C. There is insufficient research to support universal use in individuals with diabetes.

   D. Natural agents are subject to rigorous government safety and efficacy testing, so they are safe for use.

145. The manufacturer of a new blood glucose meter would like to provide free products to patients using insulin at a rural clinic. To decrease the diabetes educator's workload, the manufacturer suggests that it contact the patients directly to arrange shipment. Which of the following is the MOST appropriate response for this educator?

   A. Generate a listing of names and addresses of all patients with diabetes for the manufacturer

   B. Generate a listing of names and telephone numbers of all patients on insulin for the manufacturer

   C. Generate a letter to all patients on insulin and advise them to contact the manufacturer

   D. Generate a listing of names and addresses of all clinic patients for the manufacturer

146. A 25-year-old female college student presents to the clinic for follow-up on her insulin therapy. She currently takes 30 units of glargine insulin at bedtime and 6 units of aspart insulin with meals. She reports frequent episodes of low blood glucose before lunch during the past month. Based on the graph of blood glucose values below, which of the following therapy changes is MOST appropriate?

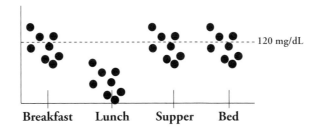

   A. Decrease bedtime glargine insulin dose to 20 units

   B. Move glargine insulin to morning and maintain current dose

   C. Decrease morning aspart insulin to 4 units

   D. Divide glargine insulin to 15 units twice daily

Review Guide for the CDE® Exam

147. Which educational theory/model aims to identify and resolve ambivalence toward behavior change?

     A. Motivational interviewing

     B. Health belief model

     C. Social cognitive theory

     D. Transtheoretical model

148. Which of the following complications is not increased among offspring of women with gestational diabetes?

     A. Neonatal hypoglycemia

     B. Shoulder dystocia

     C. Macrosomia

     D. Congenital malformations

149. Which of the following traits is the LEAST essential for effective pattern management?

     A. Problem-solving skills

     B. Health literacy

     C. Willingness to learn

     D. Sound knowledge of diabetes self-care skills and behaviors

150. Based on the Diabetes Education Algorithm, all of the following are appropriate action steps for DSMES at diagnosis EXCEPT:

     A. a review of medication choices.

     B. making a referral for medical nutrition therapy.

     C. an emphasis on risk reduction.

     D. developing personal strategies to address psychosocial issues and concerns.

Read the following vignette to answer the next 3 questions.

   CJ is a 45-year-old woman with a 10-year history of type 2 diabetes who is referred to you for instruction and initiation of insulin therapy. Her physician has given her a prescription for a prefilled 70/30 insulin pen.

151. What teaching format would you anticipate to be MOST effective?

     A. Lecture

     B. Audiovisual aids

     C. Demonstration

     D. Print materials

54

Section 3: Practice Exams

152. The patient asks you how long she can safely keep the insulin pen she is using unrefrigerated. What would you advise?

    A. 1 to 5 days

    B. 6 to 9 days

    C. 10 to 14 days

    D. 15 to 21 days

153. In talking with CJ, you realize that she is extremely resistant to the idea of taking insulin injections. When you explore her feelings further, you find out that she correlates insulin administration with her mother's leg amputation and her blindness. Which of the following methods is NOT likely to reduce CJ's fear of insulin?

    A. Establishing a trusting relationship and open communication with CJ

    B. Use of motivational interviewing techniques

    C. Explaining to CJ that noncompliance with diet and exercise for the last 10 years has resulted in the need to take insulin at this point

    D. Demonstrating the use of newer options for insulin administration such as short needles and insulin pen devices

154. Which data collection tool is most appropriate to measure the outcome of "change in A1C" following completion of a diabetes self-management education program?

    A. Survey

    B. Chart audit

    C. Telephone follow-up with participants

    D. Post-program evaluation

155. A diabetes education program boasts that 97% of its 24 patients effectively achieved their behavioral change goals. According to the PIPE model, which of the following is needed to fully evaluate this program?

    A. Performance of staff based on benchmarks

    B. Penetration into the target population

    C. Integration of multiple providers

    D. Interest in self-care behaviors

Review Guide for the CDE® Exam

156. A managed care organization asks its diabetes educators to document cost savings of their activities to the organization. Which of the following is most likely to correlate with decreased cost for the organization?

   A. Learning

   B. Health status

   C. Monitoring

   D. Healthy eating

157. A patient reports exercising for 30 minutes a day 4 times a week. Which of the following best defines the level of this self-management outcome?

   A. Immediate outcome

   B. Intermediate outcome

   C. Post-intermediate outcome

   D. Long-term outcome

158. The inclusion of family members and/or a support system in the educational process is a guiding principle of which key element of DSMES?

   A. Engagement

   B. Information sharing

   C. Care coordination

   D. Psychosocial and behavioral support

159. Which of the following is considered the leading alterable risk factor associated with the development and progression of diabetes retinopathy?

   A. Renal disease

   B. Blood pressure

   C. Age

   D. Glucose control

160. Documentation of self-management education

   A. should occur at every step in the diabetes self-management education (DSME) process.

   B. is a one-time event.

   C. should capture immediate but not long-term outcomes.

   D. is not protected by the Health Insurance Portability and Accountability Act (HIPAA).

Section 3: Practice Exams

161. A patient takes insulin glargine at bedtime and insulin glulisine at meals based on an insulin-to-carbohydrate ratio. Which of the following is the most appropriate interpretation of information from the blood glucose log of this patient?

Breakfast		Lunch		Dinner	
Before mg/dL	After mg/dL	Before mg/dL	After mg/dL	Before mg/dL	After mg/dL
95	137				
		112	140	176	
99		98	138	161	149
91		94	143	172	
100	139			163	

   A. Insulin-to-carbohydrate ratio at lunch is incorrect

   B. Insulin-to-carbohydrate ratio at breakfast is incorrect

   C. Glargine is wearing off early

   D. Experiencing dawn phenomenon

162. A patient with type 2 diabetes that is controlled by lifestyle modification reports that her typical weekday breakfast is 1/4 cup liquid egg substitute, 2 slices turkey bacon, 1 slice whole wheat toast with margarine, and 1/2 cup apple juice, and that her 2-hour postmeal blood glucose generally runs <140 mg/dL. She has noticed, however, that on Saturdays when she eats 2 pancakes with 1/4 cup of light syrup, 1/2 banana, and 1 cup skim milk, her 2-hour postmeal blood glucose runs higher. What is a reasonable explanation?

   A. Breakfast carbohydrate intake is higher on the weekend

   B. Breakfast carbohydrate intake is lower on the weekend

   C. Breakfast carbohydrate intake is equivalent at weekday and weekend meals, so physical activity must be lower on the weekends

   D. Variation in meal timing is contributing to blood glucose variation

163. The recognition of personal prejudices and biases toward other cultures is known as cultural

   A. humility.

   B. knowledge.

   C. awareness.

   D. desire.

164. Which of the following is the most effective method to determine an individual's grasp of carbohydrate counting?

   A. Ask the patient to keep a food log

   B. Have the patient calculate the carbohydrate count of a typical meal

   C. Have the patient list foods high in carbohydrate

   D. Ask the patient to read food labels and identify carbohydrate content

Review Guide for the CDE® Exam

165. Changes in physical activity levels and problem-solving abilities are good indicators of
     A. learning.
     B. continuous quality improvement.
     C. behavior change.
     D. improved health status.

166. Which of the following demonstrates progress toward achievement of a behavior goal?
     A. John has read some information about diabetes since his last appointment
     B. John monitors his blood glucose 3 times per day
     C. John can identify 4 foods that contain carbohydrate
     D. John can describe appropriate hypoglycemia treatment

167. A patient takes detemir insulin 20 units every morning and 10 units before bedtime. Based on the blood glucose log, what is the most appropriate recommendation?

Breakfast		Lunch		Dinner	
Before mg/dL	Carbs g	Before mg/dL	Carbs g	Before mg/dL	Carbs g
122	50	60	55	74	
104	55	99	60	71	
114	50	63	65	66	
110	50	65	60	73	

     A. Decrease bedtime detemir
     B. Move bedtime detemir before dinner
     C. Decrease morning detemir dose
     D. Add predinner aspart insulin

168. A pediatric endocrinologist contracts with a diabetes educator to develop a new curriculum for patients in the practice. Which of the following is the MOST appropriate consideration for this educator?
     A. Select educational material that can be read by 6-year-old children
     B. Set up the education sessions to accommodate one parent and child at a time
     C. Incorporate examples and opportunities for play as much as possible
     D. Use computerized slide presentations as the primary information delivery method

Section 3: Practice Exams

169. Which of the following oral agents is approved by the Food and Drug Administration (FDA) for use in children aged 10 years or older?

    A. Glyburide

    B. Acarbose

    C. Glipizide

    D. Metformin

170. At an initial diabetes education appointment, a patient agrees to a goal of exercising 30 minutes every day. At a 1-month follow-up visit, the patient states that he has only been able to exercise 15 minutes 4 days a week and that exercising 30 minutes every day seems overwhelming. What is an appropriate follow-up action?

    A. Continue with the original exercise goal of 30 minutes 7 days a week

    B. Adjust the exercise goal to 15 minutes 4 days a week

    C. Set an intermediate exercise goal of working up to 20 minutes 6 or 7 days a week by the 3-month follow-up appointment

    D. Discontinue exercise since the goal can't be achieved

171. A 45-year-old patient presents for an initial diabetes education evaluation. During the session, the patient states that he "forgot his glasses" and that his wife read him the background questionnaire in the waiting room. Which of the following is the MOST important consideration when developing an education plan for this patient?

    A. The educator should avoid providing any written materials

    B. The patient's wife should attend all education sessions

    C. The patient may have cognitive deficits

    D. The patient may have low literacy

172. An elderly patient with type 2 diabetes comes into the pharmacy after spending all afternoon holiday shopping at the mall. He tells you his "heart is racing" and he is sweaty and shaky. What is the best course of action for this patient?

    A. Take 4 glucose tablets and then check his blood glucose

    B. Check his blood glucose and inject NPH insulin if hyperglycemic

    C. Eat a candy bar and drink a regular soda and then check his blood glucose

    D. Check his blood glucose and call emergency services if it is normal

59

Review Guide for the CDE® Exam

173. The Food and Drug Administration (FDA) and the Centers for Disease Control and Prevention (CDC) have established infection control guidelines for the use of blood glucose monitoring devices. What is NOT included in the recommendations to reduce the risk of blood-borne pathogens in performing self-blood glucose monitoring?

    A. Clean meter and disinfect with disinfectant recommended by the manufacturer

    B. Clean and disinfect penlet-style lancing device endcap prior to using on multiple persons

    C. Dispose of lancets in an approved sharps container

    D. Lancing devices should never be used for more than one person

174. A 57-year-old patient with impaired glucose tolerance and chronic stable angina returns for diabetes education with a list of herbal products from the local health food store clerk. Which of the following is the MOST appropriate product recommendation for this patient based on the strength of supporting evidence?

    A. Cinnamon

    B. Chromium picolinate

    C. Ginseng

    D. Aspirin

175. MP reports symptoms of sweating, lack of concentration, and restlessness, but reports that her blood glucose levels are always >130 mg/dL. What diagnosis might you suspect?

    A. Anxiety disorder

    B. Depressive disorder

    C. Flu

    D. Social phobia

176. A 23-year-old female patient with type 1 diabetes visits her endocrinologist every 3 months. Which of the following is the MOST appropriate recommendation for this patient to maintain healthy vision?

    A. The endocrinologist should visually inspect the patient's eyes at each visit

    B. An ophthalmologist should perform a dilated examination annually

    C. An optometrist should evaluate the patient for corrective lenses every 3 years

    D. The endocrinologist should physically examine the patient's eyes twice yearly

177. Which of the following statements about preconception care is TRUE?

    A. It reduces risk of congenital malformations

    B. Its benefits in women with type 2 diabetes have not been determined

    C. It improves fertility

    D. It is best initiated upon confirmation of a positive pregnancy test

Section 3: Practice Exams

178. A patient presents with urinary albumin-to-creatinine ratio (UACR) of 106 mg/g and estimated glomerular filtration rate (eGFR) of 50 mL/min/1.73m². Into which stage of chronic kidney disease would this patient be classified?

    A. Stage 1

    B. Stage 2

    C. Stage 3

    D. Stage 4

179. You are seeing TK for diabetes education. She tells you that she has been feeling down and depressed. In addition, she is having difficulty falling asleep and concentrating. Which of the following is the most appropriate intervention?

    A. Reassess her symptoms at the next visit

    B. Refer to a mental health professional

    C. Refer to a stress reduction program

    D. Provide education on depression and its impact on diabetes

180. JJ, usually talkative and jovial, returns for a routine 3-month follow-up appointment. Today his lips are pursed and he sits with his arms crossed. Due to the diabetes educator's rapport with him, he soon becomes tearful and states that he and his wife are fighting again. He adds that it has been difficult to focus on managing his diabetes. What is the MOST appropriate response to JJ?

    A. Refocus the discussion on diabetes management

    B. Reschedule the appointment for another time

    C. Refer him and his wife to a marriage counselor

    D. Refer him to a psychiatrist to start an anti-depressant drug

181. A 5-year-old boy is ready for hospital discharge following initial stabilization of newly diagnosed type 1 diabetes. Initial comprehensive diabetes education has been provided. In departure discussions with the parents, the diabetes educator notes that they appear quite anxious. They state several times that they're scared and have asked what they should do if they encounter situations that they're not confident managing. Which of the following is the most appropriate response from the diabetes educator?

    A. Assure parents that they will be able to meet the challenges

    B. Tell parents that other families have overcome the challenges

    C. Refer parents to a stress reduction program

    D. Provide parents with contact information for the diabetes healthcare team

Review Guide for the CDE® Exam

182. You are seeing EW for nutrition counseling. Her clinical data are as follows: blood pressure 145/92 mm Hg, A1C 6.4%, BMI 24 kg/m², total cholesterol 260 mg/dL. What is the MOST appropriate nutrition prescription for this patient?

    A. Low carbohydrate diet

    B. DASH eating plan

    C. Low-fat diet

    D. Unrestricted diet with carbohydrate counting

183. You are conducting an evaluation of your DSME program. You wish to determine how many individuals have received a foot exam and eye exam during the past year. Which of the following data collection tools would be best utilized to meet your objective?

    A. Perform a time study

    B. Distribute a patient checklist at the last program session

    C. Perform a chart audit for all participants

    D. Conduct a phone survey of all participants during follow-up

184. A motivated individual is identified by the diabetes nurse educator as an appropriate insulin pump candidate. He monitors his blood glucose 6 times per day and has recently been keeping a food log to determine the impact of different foods and meals on his blood glucose. Currently, he's not following any meal plan. Which of the following referrals is essential before initiating an insulin pump request?

    A. Exercise physiologist for an exercise plan

    B. Registered dietitian for an 1,800-calorie meal plan

    C. Psychologist to ensure the individual is emotionally prepared for a pump

    D. Registered dietitian for carbohydrate counting

185. An 83-year-old woman on glipizide lives alone, has no family nearby, and refuses to enter assisted living. She relies on friends and neighbors to get her groceries, for which she generously pays them. Her weight has unintentionally decreased by 6 lbs since her last visit, and she experiences occasional hypoglycemia. Which of the following is the most appropriate referral for this patient?

    A. Registered dietitian

    B. Pharmacist

    C. Financial counselor

    D. Community meal program

SECTION 3:
PRACTICE EXAMS

62

Section 3: Practice Exams

186. A 41-year-old man with recently diagnosed type 2 diabetes presents for diabetes education. He complains of blurry vision and states he can't read the newspaper print. He does not wear corrective lenses and his last eye exam was 5 years ago. What is the MOST appropriate recommendation?

    A. Referral to an optometrist for a vision screening

    B. Referral to an ophthalmologist for a comprehensive dilated eye exam

    C. Advise the patient to purchase reading glasses

    D. Wait 3 months to see if vision improves; if there is no improvement, schedule an appointment for vision evaluation

Read the following vignette to answer the next 3 questions.

A 49-year-old Hispanic male presents at his primary care physician's office with fatigue, polydipsia, polyuria, and 20-lb weight loss over the past 3 weeks. He is married with 2 young children and does not have health insurance. Additional information gathered:

- Fasting blood glucose 498 mg/dL
- A1C 13.4%
- Negative serum ketones

187. What is the MOST likely diagnosis?

    A. Type 1 diabetes

    B. Diabetic ketoacidosis (DKA)

    C. Type 2 diabetes

    D. Impaired fasting glucose

188. Which of the following treatment plans is MOST appropriate for this patient?

    A. Pioglitazone

    B. Acarbose

    C. Glargine insulin

    D. Exenatide

189. Besides referral to a diabetes educator, what additional referral is most appropriate?

    A. Mental health

    B. Financial/social services

    C. Home health

    D. Cardiology

Review Guide for the CDE® Exam

190. Soliciting and responding to questions is a guiding principle of which key element of DSMES?

    A. Engagement

    B. Information sharing

    C. Psychosocial and behavioral support

    D. Care coordination

191. Participant completion of a post-survey on a diabetes self-management program provides valuable feedback on

    A. process data.

    B. lab data.

    C. learning and behavior change.

    D. the scheduling issues.

192. A 28-year-old woman with type 1 diabetes is considering becoming pregnant. She has been reading about the risks of hyperglycemia during pregnancy and is very concerned. She has decided that she wants to start checking her blood glucose more often. According to the transtheoretical model, in what stage of change is this woman?

    A. Precontemplation

    B. Contemplation

    C. Preparation

    D. Maintenance

193. Which of the following class of medications act within the intestinal wall to prevent/delay the breakdown of certain carbohydrates?

    A. Sulfonylureas

    B. Thiazolidinediones

    C. Dipeptidyl peptidase 4 (DPP-4) inhibitors

    D. Alpha-glucosidase inhibitors

194. Which of the following represents the minimum Dietary Reference Intake (DRI) of carbohydrate for pregnant women?

    A. 130 g/day

    B. 100 g/day

    C. 175 g/day

    D. 200 g/day

SECTION 3: PRACTICE EXAMS

64

Section 3: Practice Exams

195. A diabetes educator's chart note reads, "The patient and her husband own a small restaurant. They have no health insurance and $500 in medical bills from the past 2 weeks. She became tearful at the mention of purchasing a blood glucose meter and testing supplies." According to the note, the diabetes educator has assessed which of the following?

    A. Financial status

    B. Cultural beliefs

    C. Health beliefs

    D. Literacy

196. Which of the following is the most effective method to assess the injection technique of a teenager new to insulin?

    A. Parent demonstration of injection technique

    B. Parent description of injection technique by the teenager injects appropriately

    C. Teenager demonstration of injection technique

    D. Teenager description of injection technique

197. To reduce complication risk, what is the American Diabetes Association's (ADA's) A1C general goal for individuals with diabetes?

    A. <6%

    B. <7%

    C. <7.5%

    D. <8%

198. Which of the following models or theories assumes that optimal care is achieved when a prepared proactive healthcare team interacts with an informed activated patient?

    A. Chronic care model

    B. Social cognitive theory

    C. Health belief model

    D. Theory of reasoned action and planned behavior

199. An 82-year-old woman comes to the clinic alone for general diabetes education. She states that her daughter helps with the housework and her medications. Which of the following is the MOST appropriate approach for this patient?

    A. Ask the patient to take careful notes and have the daughter call with questions

    B. Telephone the woman's daughter after the visit to review material

    C. Ask if the patient would like her daughter to attend the session

    D. Provide the patient with written materials to take home

65

Review Guide for the CDE® Exam

200. According to the American Diabetes Association (ADA), peak postprandial plasma glucose levels for patients with diabetes should NOT exceed which of the following?

   A. 120 mg/dL

   B. 140 mg/dL

   C. 180 mg/dL

   D. 240 mg/dL

Exam 2

1. The single most important factor in predicting A1C lowering with the use of continuous glucose monitoring (CGM) has been shown to be which of the following?

   A. Frequency of device calibration

   B. Use of a higher low-glucose alarm setting

   C. Frequency of sensor use

   D. Age of the patient using the device

2. Which of the following islet cell antibodies is the best immunologic predictor of type 1 diabetes?

   A. Glutamic acid decarboxylase (GAD)

   B. Heat shock protein 65

   C. Peripherin

   D. Endocrine cell antigens

3. A thin 38-year-old white female presents to the clinic for evaluation of her glycemic control. She was diagnosed with diabetes 9 months ago with an A1C of 13% and started on metformin and glipizide. Three months later her glycemic control was much improved (A1C of 7.4%), but today she reports increased thirst and urination. Her A1C today is 11.2% despite confirmed adherence with her medications and a negative pregnancy test. Which of the following is the MOST likely diagnosis?

   A. Type 1 diabetes (T1DM)

   B. Type 2 diabetes (T2DM)

   C. Latent autoimmune diabetes of adults (LADA)

   D. Gestational diabetes (GDM)

Section 3: Practice Exams

4. The development of type 1 diabetes includes all but which of the following?

    A. Environmental trigger

    B. Genetic predisposition

    C. Autoimmune attack on beta cells

    D. Peripheral insulin resistance

5. JT, a 34-year-old male with newly diagnosed type 1 diabetes and hypertension, states that he has an occasional alcoholic drink and wants to know if alcohol is allowed. Which of the following is the MOST appropriate response?

    A. Yes, but always consume alcohol with food to minimize the risk of nocturnal hypoglycemia

    B. It is recommended to drink 2 glasses of red wine every day to reduce the risk of cardiovascular disease

    C. Yes, but substitute an alcoholic drink for 1 carb serving

    D. No, alcoholic beverages should be avoided in persons with hypertension due to the impact on blood pressure

6. A 45-year-old man presents for a 1-month follow-up after starting immediate release metformin 500 mg twice daily. Today he brought in his blood glucose meter and bottle of metformin, which is nearly full. Which of the following is the MOST appropriate next step to evaluate his adherence to the regimen?

    A. Confront the patient about his noncompliance

    B. Telephone the pharmacy to verify the last refill date

    C. Change to the extended release formulation of metformin

    D. Review self-monitored blood glucose log

7. You receive an inquiry from a fellow healthcare professional in your facility who would like to use an app on her smartphone to track calories, carbohydrate, and fat consumed. She asks you how much carbohydrate and fat a person with type 2 diabetes should consume in her diet. Based on current recommendations from the American Diabetes Association (ADA), which of the following is the best advice?

    A. Persons with diabetes should get about 50% of their calories from carbohydrate and no more than 30% of calories from fat

    B. The ideal percentage of carbohydrate, protein, and fat has not been determined and is based on several factors

    C. Persons with diabetes should get about 45% of calories from carbohydrate and 25% to 30% of calories from fat

    D. A monounsaturated fat–rich eating plan with less than 25% of calories from fat and 50% to 60% of calories from carbohydrate is recommended for persons with diabetes

Review Guide for the CDE® Exam

8. A 48-year-old African American woman with type 2 diabetes and hypertension presents to the clinic accompanied by her mother, who stays in the waiting room during the visit. The patient lives at home and does not work. She reports attending community college for 2 years but has never held a full-time job. Answers to questions during the interview are disorganized and rambling with frequent flights of thought. Which of the following is the MOST appropriate action to evaluate this patient?

    A. Interview the patient alone and make changes based on objective data

    B. Engage the patient in role-playing to evaluate problem-solving skills

    C. Ask permission from the patient to include her mother in the visit

    D. Contact the mother after the visit to express mental health concerns

9. According to the American Diabetes Association's (ADA's) current Guidelines, A1C testing should be performed at least _____ in patients who are meeting treatment goals.

    A. once/year

    B. twice/year

    C. every 3 months

    D. every 4 months

Use the following scenario to answer the next 3 questions.

> AE is a 45-year-old obese female with uncontrolled type 2 diabetes (A1C 8.5%), hypertriglyceridemia (425 mg/dL), and hypertension (145/90). She has a sedentary job as a receptionist. Her usual diet includes a bagel with cream cheese or grits, eggs, toast, and coffee at the cafeteria at work, a fast-food burger or Mexican food at lunch, snack bar or nuts as snacks, and takeout from a local restaurant for dinner. Evening snack is often sweets. She does not drink alcoholic beverages. She does not feel she has time to exercise as she has a long commute to work and gets home late.

10. AE would like to reduce her blood pressure without using medication as she is concerned about the side effects. What would be the most appropriate recommendation for this patient?

    A. Start drinking a glass of red wine every day

    B. Follow the DASH eating plan

    C. Use sea salt or kosher salt in place of table salt

    D. Join a gym and begin a resistance training program at least 5x/week

11. Considering AE's problem list, what 2 behavioral goals would likely be the MOST important to focus on initially in AE's diet?

    A. Counting calories and counting carbs

    B. Choosing healthier options at fast-food restaurants and following an exchange diet

    C. Consuming less saturated fats and using less added salt

    D. Counting carbs and eating out less frequently

Section 3: Practice Exams

12. What is the most appropriate evidence-based advice for AE regarding her sodium intake?

    A. Reducing the amount of salt one uses at the table by 50% can lower blood pressure significantly

    B. A combination of following the DASH dietary pattern and reducing sodium intake has been shown to lower blood pressure more than simply reducing sodium intake alone

    C. About 45% of sodium intake comes from processed foods

    D. The American Diabetes Association (ADA) recommends that persons with diabetes reduce their sodium intake to less than 1,500 mg/day

13. According to the Diabetes Prevention Program (DPP), which of the following was MOST effective for preventing diabetes?

    A. Intensive lifestyle modifications

    B. Metformin

    C. Acarbose

    D. Rosiglitazone

14. A homeless patient presents to the clinic for evaluation of his insulin regimen. He reports riding his bicycle to the clinic, which is located 3 blocks from the discount pharmacy. He generally only eats 1 meal a day in the evening at the shelter. This afternoon his point-of-care blood glucose is 286 mg/dL, which is higher than his A1C level of 7.6% would suggest. Which of the following is the MOST likely cause of his elevated blood glucose?

    A. Lack of transportation to the pharmacy

    B. Inability to pay for insulin

    C. Irregular meal schedule

    D. Multiple use of the same syringe

15. Which of the following most appropriately describes the mechanisms of action for liraglutide?

    A. Increases glucagon release from alpha-cells

    B. Decreases centrally mediated satiety

    C. Increases insulin secretion from beta-cells

    D. Decreases absorption of complex carbohydrates

16. Which of the following is NOT an evidence-based recommendation for individuals managing hypertension?

    A. Weight loss for overweight or obese persons

    B. Sodium reduction

    C. Resistance training

    D. DASH eating plan

69

Review Guide for the CDE® Exam

17. Which of the following lifestyle strategies is LEAST effective in reducing LDL-cholesterol?

    A. Weight loss

    B. Substitution of mono- and polyunsaturated fats for saturated fats

    C. Omega-3 fatty acids

    D. Consumption of foods fortified with plant sterol and stanols

18. A patient had routine laboratory levels drawn 1 month after changing therapy. His serum creatinine rose from 0.9 mg/dL at baseline to 1.5 mg/dL today. Which of the following drugs MOST likely explains this rise in serum creatinine?

    A. Metoprolol

    B. Atorvastatin

    C. Metformin

    D. Irbesartan

19. A local church leader wants to offer a program to prevent diabetes. The members of the church are predominantly African American with an average age of 54. Which of the following recommendations is MOST appropriate for the members?

    A. Fast 3 days per week

    B. Walk 150 minutes per week

    C. Eat 7 servings of fatty fish per week

    D. Advise the leader that his population is low risk

20. The American Diabetes Association uses a classification system to grade the quality of scientific evidence to support its recommendations in all new and revised position statements. The highest level of evidence is rated as which of the following?

    A. A

    B. B

    C. C

    D. E

21. An obese 32-year-old patient with type 2 diabetes expresses interest in losing weight. She returns 1 month after starting her new diet and is disappointed that she gained 5 lbs. She reports eliminating all fried and fast foods. She eats 2 bananas every day and drinks 12 ounces of fruit juice with each meal. Which of the following is the best advice for this patient?

    A. Increase exercise to 300 minutes per week to burn fat

    B. Eliminate bananas from the diet due to calorie density

    C. Switch from fruit juice to water to avoid excess calories

    D. Add fried foods back to the diet to increase metabolism

70

Section 3: Practice Exams

22. ST is a 67-year-old female who reports that she is frequently waking up in the morning with a headache and has noticed that she is having more nightmares than usual. She was started on 20 units of 70/30 insulin before breakfast and dinner at her last visit. Which of the following is the MOST likely cause of the patient's problem?

    A. Dawn effect

    B. Menopause

    C. Late-night snacking

    D. Middle-of-the-night hypoglycemia

23. What nutrient is MOST likely to be deficient without supplementation or fortification in a vegan-style eating plan?

    A. Vitamin C

    B. Protein

    C. Niacin

    D. Vitamin B12

24. A 45-year-old patient with type 1 diabetes reports several hypoglycemic episodes over the past 20 years requiring hospitalization. He currently takes glargine every morning and lispro before main meals. His A1C is 8.2% with fasting blood glucose of 250 mg/dL. He reports eating 3 meals daily with a large bedtime snack for which he does not bolus. Which of the following is the MOST likely reason for his resistance to taking insulin before the bedtime snack?

    A. Fear of insulin antibodies

    B. Fear of multiple injections

    C. Fear of nocturnal hypoglycemia

    D. Fear of increasing insulin resistance

25. Which of the following represents the American Diabetes Association's (ADA's) recommendation for fiber intake for individuals with diabetes?

    A. 25 grams per day for women and 38 grams per day for men

    B. 30 grams of dietary fiber per day for both men and women

    C. 35 grams per day for women and 48 grams per day for men

    D. 50 grams of dietary fiber per day for both men and women

SECTION 3: PRACTICE EXAMS

Review Guide for the CDE® Exam

26. A 57-year-old man with coronary artery disease, type 2 diabetes, and hypertension presents to the clinic. His current medications include metformin, hydrochlorothiazide, and metoprolol. His A1C is 7.5% and his blood pressure is 150/92 mmHg. Which of the following medications would be the MOST appropriate addition to prevent microvascular complications?

    A. Gabapentin

    B. Simvastatin

    C. Valsartan

    D. Aspirin

27. Which of the following mean plasma glucose levels corresponds to an A1C of 8.0%?

    A. 154 mg/dL

    B. 183 mg/dL

    C. 212 mg/dL

    D. 240 mg/dL

28. Evidence suggests that dietary fiber

    A. may improve glycemia in amounts >50 g/day.

    B. has no benefit on serum cholesterol levels.

    C. intake in the United States is about 30 g/day.

    D. significantly lowers HDL cholesterol.

29. A 63-year-old man with coronary artery disease, type 2 diabetes, and hypertension presents to the clinic. Which of the following would be the MOST appropriate antiplatelet recommendation to reduce the risk of macrovascular complications?

    A. Aspirin 81 mg daily

    B. Aspirin 325 mg daily

    C. Clopidogrel 75 mg daily

    D. Warfarin 5 mg daily

30. Current nutrition guidelines from the American Diabetes Association (ADA) for individuals with diabetes include which of the following?

    A. Limit cholesterol to <300 mg, saturated fat to <10%, and limit *trans* fat as much as possible

    B. Limit total fat to <30% of calories, saturated fat to <8%, and limit *trans* fat as much as possible

    C. Limit cholesterol to <200 mg, saturated fat to <8%, and *trans* fat as much as possible

    D. Limit cholesterol to <200 mg, saturated fat to <10%, and avoid *trans* fats

Section 3: Practice Exams

31. A 37-year-old woman with a fasting plasma glucose of 115 mg/dL and blood pressure of 138/88 mmHg presents to the clinic. Which of the following would be necessary to diagnose this patient with metabolic syndrome?

    A. Body mass index (BMI) >30

    B. Waist circumference >35 inches

    C. Family history of diabetes

    D. LDL cholesterol >190 mg/dL

32. According to the American Diabetes Association's (ADA's) Standards of Care, which of the following characteristics justifies more stringent efforts to lower A1C?

    A. Absence of comorbidities and vascular complications

    B. Limited resources and social support

    C. Long-standing diabetes

    D. High risk for hypoglycemia

33. Which of the following is NOT included in the DASH eating plan?

    A. Low-fat dairy

    B. Emphasis on fruits and vegetables

    C. Reduced in red meat

    D. Low in carbohydrate

34. Which of the following is MOST likely to occur in patients with type 2 diabetes?

    A. Decreased hepatic gluconeogenesis

    B. Increased synthesis of beta cells

    C. Decreased release of glucagon

    D. Decreased release of incretins

35. Jane has questions about the heart-protective effects from omega-3 fatty acids. Which of the following would be the best recommendation for Jane?

    A. Start taking 1,000–3,000 mg/d of omega-3 fatty acid supplements

    B. Eat at least 2 servings of only wild-caught fish per week

    C. Supplement her diet with alfalfa sprouts, chia seeds, and flaxseed oil

    D. Eat at least 2 servings of fatty fish per week

73

Review Guide for the CDE® Exam

36. Self-monitoring of blood glucose (SMBG) should be performed more frequently in which of the following situations?

    A. Presence of intercurrent illness

    B. During preconception and pregnancy

    C. To manage hypoglycemia unawareness

    D. All of the above

37. A 63-year-old woman with type 2 diabetes complains of a corn on her right foot. The skin on her left foot is intact, but she is missing 2 toes due to a previous amputation. Her A1C is 11.5% on insulin plus metformin. In addition to her other medicines, she also takes gabapentin for peripheral neuropathy. What is the MOST appropriate foot care advice for this patient?

    A. Apply rubbing alcohol to her feet twice a day

    B. Encourage her to consult with a local podiatrist

    C. Refer her to a pharmacist to select a corn remover

    D. Soak her feet in warm water and then use a scalpel to cut away the corn

38. A provider calls the diabetes educator asking for clarification about pen needles for a lean patient with type 1 diabetes. Which of the following recommendations is most appropriate?

    A. 4-mm needles are reserved for children

    B. 5-mm length needles are intended for use on arms or thighs

    C. 6-mm length needles may be used without pinching a skinfold

    D. 12.7-mm length needles may be used without pinching a skinfold

Use the following scenario to answer the next 4 questions.

MA is a 32-year-old female with new-onset type 2 diabetes. Her A1C is 8.5% and her BMI 31. She is very sedentary in her work as a receptionist in a small business. She appears somewhat overwhelmed with the diagnosis of diabetes and states that she doesn't have much time to devote to managing it.

39. Which of the following agents would be most useful for MA to lose weight?

    A. Pioglitazone

    B. Dulaglutide

    C. Glimepiride

    D. Nateglinide

Section 3: Practice Exams

40. What is the minimal amount of information on the food label that MA would need to count carbohydrate to avoid complexity and confusion?

   A. Sugars and total carbohydrate

   B. Serving size and total carbohydrate

   C. Total carbohydrate, sugars, and sugar alcohols

   D. Serving size and sugars

41. From the following list, which nutrition tool would be the best choice to use to teach MA about basic carbohydrate counting?

   A. The Mediterranean Eating Plan

   B. Choose Your Foods: Food Lists for Diabetes

   C. Count Your Carbs: Getting Started

   D. DASH eating plan

42. MA set her goals to consume about 3 carbohydrate choices (or servings) per meal and 1 choice at her evening snack. How many grams of carbohydrate should she have at each meal?

   A. 15 grams

   B. 30 grams

   C. 45 grams

   D. 60 grams

43. Upon physical exam of a 35-year-old obese woman, a physician notices dark pigmented skin around her neck. The physician identifies the area as acanthosis nigricans. Which of the following best describes the hyperpigmentation cause in this patient?

   A. Poor hygiene

   B. Insulin resistance

   C. Genetic predisposition

   D. Metformin adverse effect

44. Which of the following scenarios would be a reason to use control solution to evaluate the accuracy of blood glucose (BG) meter results?

   A. Using the wrong code on the meter

   B. Applying an inadequate sample of blood

   C. Leaving the cap off the vial of strips

   D. Not washing hands prior to performing self-monitoring of blood glucose (SMBG)

Review Guide for the CDE® Exam

45. The Mediterranean diet is characterized by which of the following?

    A. Limited alcohol consumption

    B. High consumption of milk and dairy products

    C. High ratio of monounsaturated to saturated fats

    D. Low consumption of nonrefined cereals and legumes

46. A patient with type 2 diabetes noticed a 15-lb weight gain over the past 2 years. Which of the following drugs would MOST likely worsen her weight gain?

    A. Pramlintide

    B. Exenatide

    C. Pioglitazone

    D. Saxagliptin

47. LL is a 47-year-old female on 1,000 mg metformin twice a day. Her A1C is 7.5% and her BMI is 33. LL spends most of her time at work on a computer and is very sedentary outside work. She does little cooking and eats in restaurants frequently. What would be the major benefit of self-monitoring of blood glucose (SMBG) for LL at this time?

    A. Provide information for titration of metformin

    B. Detect, identify, and prevent hypoglycemia

    C. Facilitate behavior change

    D. Determine the need for insulin

48. An overweight 38-year-old woman with type 2 diabetes is motivated to lose weight. In addition to lifestyle interventions, which of the following is the best treatment recommendation for this patient?

    A. Glyburide

    B. Detemir

    C. Saxagliptin

    D. Liraglutide

49. Which of the following does not affect the accuracy of A1C tests?

    A. Sickle cell anemia

    B. Iron deficiency

    C. Iron supplementation

    D. Low albumin

Section 3: Practice Exams

50. What is the typical lipid profile of individuals with prediabetes?

    A. High HDL, low triglycerides, and LDL may be elevated, borderline, or normal

    B. Low HDL, LDL, and triglycerides

    C. Elevated LDL, with normal levels of HDL and triglycerides

    D. Low HDL, elevated triglycerides, and LDL may be elevated, borderline, or normal

51. A 65-year-old retired chemistry professor states that he is frustrated by his continued poor glycemic control. He currently takes metformin twice daily and eats 3 meals a day. His 3-day food diary reveals pastries for breakfast, cake after lunch, and a large bowl of ice cream after dinner. Which of the following best describes the poor understanding about the relationship between food and glycemic control in this patient?

    A. Numeracy

    B. Literacy

    C. Education level

    D. Health literacy

52. Discrepancies between the average self-monitoring of blood glucose (SMBG) results from a meter and the A1C may be due to all but which of the following?

    A. Checking BG results only prebreakfast and predinner

    B. Comparing the 90-day meter average with an A1C

    C. Meter inaccuracy

    D. Incorrect SMBG technique

53. A 42-year-old patient with type 2 diabetes on metformin 1,000 mg twice daily presents for evaluation. His A1C is 7.8% despite excellent compliance with his metformin, diet, and exercise recommendations. His health insurance supplements his gym membership and he would like to "lose a few more pounds." Which of the following would be the best option for this active patient?

    A. Dapagliflozin

    B. Glipizide

    C. Pioglitazone

    D. Glargine

54. Which of the following characterizes the normal hormonal response during acute physical activity?

    A. Decreased insulin and increased glucagon and epinephrine

    B. Increased insulin, glucagon, and epinephrine

    C. Decreased insulin, glucagon, and epinephrine

    D. Increased insulin, glucagon, and cortisol

Review Guide for the CDE® Exam

55. JG has type 2 diabetes and is a landscape worker in south Florida. His self-monitoring of blood glucose (SMBG) checks are performed twice daily pre- and postmeal at alternate meals. His educator notes that his results look very good for a period of time but then seem to vary widely from his A1C. Which of the following would be the MOST likely cause of inaccurate results from his SMBG?

    A. Improper calibration

    B. Improper storage of strips

    C. Expired strips

    D. Inaccurate meter

56. To reduce the risk of hypoglycemia in a patient with type 1 diabetes, a snack containing _____ grams of carbohydrate should be consumed for every 30 to 45 minutes of moderate physical activity.

    A. 5 to 10

    B. 10 to 30

    C. 30 to 45

    D. 45 to 60

57. An obese elderly female patient with type 2 diabetes complains of urinary frequency, urgency, and dysuria. Her medications include canagliflozin, metformin, amlodipine, and atorvastatin. Today her A1C is 6.8% and her plasma blood glucose is 114 mg/dL. Which of the following would be the MOST likely cause of her symptoms?

    A. Poor glycemic control

    B. Metformin side effect

    C. Increased caffeine intake

    D. Canagliflozin side effect

58. JK is a 23-year-old female who is at 30 weeks' gestation and was recently diagnosed with gestational diabetes. She is referred for diabetes education and to learn self-monitoring of blood glucose (SMBG). Which of the following SMBG regimens would be MOST beneficial to reduce her risk of pregnancy-related complications?

    A. Monitor premeal

    B. Monitor fasting

    C. Monitor 1 hour postmeal

    D. Monitor 2 hours postmeal

78

Section 3: Practice Exams

59. Which of the following symptoms is NOT associated with hypoglycemia?

    A. Hunger

    B. Agitation

    C. Weakness

    D. Bradycardia

60. Alternate site testing (AST) should be avoided in persons at risk for hypoglycemia in which of the following situations?

    A. In persons using insulin sensitizers

    B. When the glucose is likely to change rapidly

    C. Before meals

    D. 2 hours after meals

61. A 22-year-old patient with type 1 diabetes checks her blood glucose at 11:00 AM after skipping breakfast. Her blood glucose level is 68 mg/dL, and she reports feeling jittery and weak. Which of the following would be the best recommendation for this patient?

    A. Inject glucagon 1 mg subcutaneously

    B. Eat something with 30 to 60 g of protein

    C. Consume tablets with 15 to 20 g of glucose

    D. Call 911 and transport to nearest hospital

62. Which of the following is NOT a factor that can affect self-monitoring of blood glucose (SMBG) accuracy in many types of meters?

    A. Temperature

    B. Polycythemia

    C. Variations in hematocrit

    D. Ibuprofen

63. DK, a 23-year-old with type 1 diabetes and a history of proliferative retinopathy, meets with the diabetes educator because he wishes to start an exercise program. Which of the following activities would be most appropriate for this patient?

    A. Weight lifting

    B. Jogging

    C. Competitive sports

    D. Swimming

Review Guide for the CDE® Exam

64. A 45-year-old patient with type 2 diabetes taking metformin 500 mg once daily presents for evaluation. His A1C today is 6.5% and he reports good compliance without any side effects. He recently purchased a new blood glucose meter and asks about testing frequency. Which of the following is the best recommendation for this patient?

    A. Test once weekly at different times

    B. Test 15 minutes after the largest meal daily

    C. Test 4 times daily before meals and at bedtime

    D. Test only if signs or symptoms of hypoglycemia occur

65. While the majority of blood glucose meters currently on the market do not require coding, there are still some meters that do require coding. Which of the following statements is TRUE about coding blood glucose meters?

    A. Incorrect coding can increase the risk of hypoglycemia in insulin-treated patients

    B. None of the meters currently on the market require coding

    C. The accuracy of no-code meters is significantly lower than the accuracy of meters requiring coding

    D. Coding a meter is used to determine the accuracy of a meter

66. A 28-year-old patient with poorly controlled type 1 diabetes presents for follow-up. Her A1C three months ago was 9.2%. Which of the following is the best recommendation regarding repeat testing of her A1C?

    A. Repeat A1C monthly until less than 7%

    B. Repeat A1C today and every 3 months thereafter

    C. Repeat A1C after home blood glucose levels are <180 mg/dL

    D. Repeat A1C every 12 months regardless of blood glucose levels

67. An 83-year-old female with type 2 diabetes has just been admitted to a skilled nursing facility (SNF). Based on the current Centers for Disease Control and Prevention (CDC) safety guidelines for the prevention of transmission of blood-borne pathogens, which of the following statements is correct regarding the use of blood glucose monitoring equipment in a multi-patient setting?

    A. Penlet-style lancing devices can be used on multiple patients as long as the end cap is changed prior to each use

    B. Blood glucose meters can be used with multiple patients if cleaned with a 70% alcohol solution after each use

    C. Only single-use auto-disabling lancets should be used in a multi-patient setting

    D. Lancing devices with cartridges containing multiple pre-loaded lancets can be designated for multi-patient use as long as a new lancet is advanced for each patient

80

Section 3: Practice Exams

68. A 62-year-old woman presents to the clinic after recently being diagnosed with type 2 diabetes. Her past medical history is significant for hypertension, chronic kidney disease, and osteoporosis. She reports walking 2 miles daily without chest pain or shortness of breath. Her laboratory values are as follows: A1C 7.6%, serum creatinine 1.8 mg/dL, microalbumin 1,326 mcg/mg. Which of the following conditions is the MOST compelling reason to avoid metformin in this patient?

    A. Unstable heart failure

    B. Renal dysfunction

    C. Osteoporosis

    D. Age >60 years old

69. In which of the following cases should glycemic goals be individualized to a higher range than the general goals by the American Diabetes Association (ADA)?

    A. Pregnancy in a woman with type 2 diabetes

    B. Stable blood glucose in a 24-year-old male with type 1 diabetes

    C. Preconception

    D. History of severe hypoglycemia

70. A patient recently started orlistat for weight loss. Which of the following should this patient avoid to minimize drug-food interactions with orlistat?

    A. Fat

    B. Sodium

    C. Potassium

    D. Sucrose

Use the following scenario to answer the next 3 questions.

You are seeing MT, a 25-year-old female with type 1 diabetes, in the office for insulin pump training. MT is carbohydrate counting, her current A1C is 8%, and her total daily insulin dose is 32 units.

71. Which of the following is the most appropriate basal rate for this patient?

    A. 0.3 units per hour

    B. 0.5 units per hour

    C. 0.7 units per hour

    D. 0.9 units per hour

81

Review Guide for the CDE® Exam

72. Which of the following represents her insulin-to-carbohydrate ratio (ICR)?

    A. 1:8
    B. 1:10
    C. 1:12
    D. 1:15

73. Which of the following represents her correction dose, the amount that 1 unit of insulin will decrease the blood glucose?

    A. 25 mg/dL
    B. 50 mg/dL
    C. 75 mg/dL
    D. 100 mg/dL

74. More frequent self-monitoring of blood glucose (SMBG) is warranted in certain situations where either safety is a concern or the information is required to help guide therapy. In which of the following scenarios would additional monitoring be warranted?

    A. Before taking a bolus based on an elevated glucose value from a continuous glucose monitor in a patient taking acetaminophen for pain
    B. Prior to exercise by an individual with type 2 diabetes being treated with a GLP-1 as monotherapy
    C. Before going to bed after a physically active day by an individual with type 2 diabetes managed with nutrition therapy
    D. Prior to driving by an individual with type 2 diabetes on metformin as monotherapy

75. Which of the following agents should be avoided in patients taking lorcaserin for weight loss?

    A. Atorvastatin
    B. Metformin
    C. Fluoxetine
    D. Lisinopril

76. Paired testing (monitoring pre- and postmeal at the same meal) is beneficial for all the following reasons EXCEPT to

    A. determine basal insulin needs.
    B. evaluate the effect of medication targeted to postprandial hyperglycemia.
    C. help determine insulin-to-carbohydrate (I:CHO) ratios.
    D. help evaluate the glycemic effect of a meal.

SECTION 3: PRACTICE EXAMS

82

Section 3: Practice Exams

77. A patient recently diagnosed with type 2 diabetes just received a new prescription for metformin. Which of the following is the MOST appropriate advice to avoid gastrointestinal side effects?

    A. Take with food or milk

    B. Take entire daily dose at bedtime

    C. Take on an empty stomach every morning

    D. Take with water only and remain upright for 30 minutes

78. SW is an obese 47-year-old male with type 2 diabetes treated with 1,000 mg metformin twice a day and 120 mg repaglinide before meals. His self-monitoring of blood glucose (SMBG) log reveals a fairly consistent carbohydrate intake and a pattern of low blood glucose values post-lunch. What change would be most appropriate for SW?

    A. Lower the dose of repaglinide prior to lunch

    B. Lower the morning dose of metformin

    C. Add a snack mid-afternoon

    D. Lower the afternoon dose of metformin

79. A frail 82-year-old Caucasian female on no prescription medications presents for evaluation of her glycemic control. Her geriatrician identified an A1C goal of 8% for this patient due to her poor health and recent osteoporotic hip fracture. Her blood pressure today is 118/60 mmHg, she is 5'4", she weighs 132 lbs, her A1C is 8.8%, and her serum creatinine is 1.5 mg/dL (estimated creatinine clearance of 27 mL/min). Which of the following drug therapy options would be MOST appropriate for this patient to reach her glycemic goal?

    A. Metformin

    B. Linagliptin

    C. Pioglitazone

    D. Canagliflozin

80. Which of the following autoimmune disorders is NOT associated with type 1 diabetes?

    A. Hashimoto thyroiditis

    B. Vitiligo

    C. Celiac sprue

    D. Inflammatory bowel disease

SECTION 3: PRACTICE EXAMS

Review Guide for the CDE® Exam

81. MF is a 66-year-old female recently diagnosed with type 2 diabetes and started on metformin. Her diabetes educator has recommended that she monitor her blood glucose levels twice daily. She has Medicare Part B and wonders if that will cover her meter and strips. You tell her that if she uses a pharmacy or mail-order supplier enrolled in Medicare, it covers 80% of the following based on NOT using insulin (after she meets her deductible):

    A. All her diabetes supplies

    B. A meter and 100 strips per month

    C. The meter and not the strips

    D. A meter and 100 strips every 3 months

82. A patient presents to the diabetes education program. She has an extensive family history of cancer (mother with breast cancer, father with prostate cancer, sister with a brain tumor). Which of the following drugs has the lowest associated cancer risk?

    A. Pioglitazone

    B. Liraglutide

    C. Sitagliptin

    D. Glipizide

83. JC has type 1 diabetes and does not perform self-monitoring of blood glucose (SMBG) after meals as recommended by her diabetes educator. You learn that the pain involved with SMBG is her reason for infrequent monitoring. Which of the following is NOT a recommended option to help her overcome this obstacle?

    A. Use the sides of the fingertips with fewer nerve endings

    B. Switch to alternate site testing

    C. Use a thinner gauge lancet and change it more frequently

    D. Use a lancing device with multiple puncture depth settings

84. A 54-year-old with coronary artery disease (CAD), hypertension, and type 2 diabetes presents to the pharmacy with a new prescription for tadalafil for erectile dysfunction from his primary care provider. His current medications include metformin, metoprolol, lisinopril, hydrochlorothiazide, and isosorbide mononitrate. He also carries sublingual nitroglycerin with him to treat chest pain. Which of the following is the MOST appropriate response from the pharmacist?

    A. Suggest that he try yohimbine before filling the prescription

    B. Advise him that vardenafil is more effective and offer to call his physician

    C. Refuse to fill the prescription and suggest that he seek marriage counseling first

    D. Advise him that tadalafil is contraindicated with nitrates and contact his physician

Section 3: Practice Exams

85. Which of the following supplements is safest for long-term use?

    A. Vitamin E

    B. EPA and DHA

    C. Vitamin C

    D. Carotene

86. Which of the following is the American Diabetes Association's (ADA's) preferred treatment for self-management of hypoglycemia?

    A. Eat carbohydrate-containing food until symptoms resolve

    B. Consume 10 grams of carbohydrate-containing food along with a source of protein

    C. Consume 15–20 grams of carbohydrate that contains glucose

    D. Administer glucagon

87. A 57-year-old patient with type 2 diabetes on NPH insulin twice daily presents to the clinic after spending all afternoon holiday shopping at the mall. She tells you that her "heart is racing" and she is nauseated, sweaty, and shaky. Which of the following is the MOST appropriate recommendation for this patient?

    A. Eat a candy bar followed by a small, high-protein meal

    B. Inject an additional dose of NPH at half of the usual amount

    C. Check her blood glucose and treat hypoglycemia if present

    D. Chew and swallow 2 or 3 glucose tablets and then eat a protein-containing snack

88. Which of the following statements about diabetic retinopathy is TRUE?

    A. Optimal control of both glucose levels and blood pressure will slow the progression of retinopathy

    B. Blurry vision is the most common symptom of early proliferative retinopathy

    C. Neovascularization is characteristic of significant macular edema

    D. Weight lifting and jogging are preferred activities for individuals with active diabetic retinopathy

89. CJ is a 17-year-old male with type 1 diabetes on a basal/bolus regimen. Self-monitoring of blood glucose (SMBG) reveals a pattern of hyperglycemia post-breakfast, although he frequently becomes hypoglycemic when he increases his insulin lispro at breakfast. He currently takes his lispro at the time he eats breakfast, and reports never missing doses. Which of the following would be the best choice to resolve this issue?

    A. Suggest taking pre-breakfast lispro earlier

    B. Suggest CJ add a mid-morning snack

    C. Suggest increasing his basal insulin

    D. Suggest CJ exercise daily either before or after breakfast

SECTION 3: PRACTICE EXAMS

85

Review Guide for the CDE® Exam

90. A 44-year-old patient with type 2 diabetes on metformin 1 g twice daily also takes glargine 40 units at bedtime. His fasting blood glucose is 210 mg/dL. Which of the following represents the MOST appropriate glargine dose change?

    A. Decrease to 36 units

    B. Increase to 41 units

    C. Increase to 46 units

    D. Move glargine to morning at current dose

91. Based on the current Standards of Medical Care in Diabetes, what is the American Diabetes Association's (ADA's) recommended premeal blood glucose target for a nonpregnant adult with diabetes?

    A. 70–120 mg/dL

    B. 70–130 mg/dL

    C. 80–120 mg/dL

    D. 80–130 mg/dL

92. A 57-year-old patient presents to the clinic for follow-up on his blood pressure on lisinopril 40 mg daily plus hydrochlorothiazide 25 mg daily. Today his blood pressure remains above his goal of less than 140/90 mmHg. Which of the following anti-hypertensive agents would be MOST appropriate to add next?

    A. Amlodipine

    B. Doxazosin

    C. Furosemide

    D. Hydralazine

93. Based on the current Standards of Medical Care in Diabetes, which of the following is included in the recommendations to increase the level of physical activity in individuals with diabetes?

    A. Perform resistance training at least 150 minutes per week

    B. Limit sedentary time by breaking up extended amounts of time (>90 minutes) spent sitting

    C. Perform weight training once/week with 15–20 repetitions per muscle group

    D. Perform 150 minutes per week of vigorous physical activity

Section 3: Practice Exams

94. Which of the following is the most appropriate recommendation for a patient with hypertension and diabetic nephropathy?

    A. Blood pressure treatment should include an ACE inhibitor

    B. Dietary protein intake should be maintained at 1 g/kg/day

    C. A1C goals should be relaxed to greater than 8%

    D. Combination of ACE inhibitors with ARBs preserve kidney function

95. A 48-year-old male patient with type 2 diabetes, hypertension, and history of myocardial infarction presents to the clinic for evaluation of his cholesterol. Based on this presentation, which of the following would be the MOST appropriate therapy?

    A. Pravastatin 20 mg

    B. Fluvastatin 20 mg

    C. Rosuvastatin 20 mg

    D. Lovastatin 20 mg

96. Which of the following is a TRUE statement about sugar alcohols/polyols?

    A. They have no effect on blood glucose levels

    B. They contain more calories than other carbohydrates

    C. When adjusting mealtime insulin, only half the grams of sugar alcohols (if >5 g) need to be counted

    D. There is strong evidence to show that the use of sugar alcohols results in weight loss

97. A 56-year-old male with type 2 diabetes, coronary artery disease (CAD), and hypercholesterolemia presents for follow-up on simvastatin 20 mg daily. Today his fasting lipid panel reveals non-HDL cholesterol of 147, triglyceride 108 mg/dL, and LDL cholesterol of 115 mg/dL. He has tried atorvastatin 20 mg daily in the past and developed myalgias. Which of the following is the best recommendation to achieve his goal of non-HDL cholesterol less than 100 or LDL cholesterol less than 70 mg/dL?

    A. Add fish oil 4 g daily

    B. Increase to simvastatin 80 mg daily

    C. Add fenofibrate 145 mg daily

    D. Switch to rosuvastatin 20 mg daily

Review Guide for the CDE® Exam

98. Advanced carbohydrate counting is a meal planning approach that would be MOST beneficial in which of the following individuals?

   A. An obese 43-year-old recently diagnosed with type 2 diabetes

   B. A 64-year-old with type 2 diabetes on a fixed insulin regimen

   C. A 28-year-old with type 2 diabetes on mixed insulin twice a day with low literacy and low numeracy skills

   D. A 31-year-old on an insulin pump who checks her blood glucose at least 5 times a day

99. Which of the following insulin products has the shortest onset of action?

   A. NPH

   B. Detemir

   C. Lispro

   D. Regular

100. Which of the following does NOT influence the glycemic effect of a food?

   A. Fiber content

   B. Ripeness

   C. Cooking time

   D. Sodium content

101. Which of the following statements about peripheral neuropathy is TRUE?

   A. Individuals with type 2 diabetes should be screened for diabetic neuropathy at diagnosis and every 3 years thereafter

   B. Strict glycemic control has been shown to prevent the development of neuropathy in patients with type 1 diabetes

   C. Electrophysiological testing should always be performed to establish the diagnosis of peripheral neuropathy

   D. Effective treatments for neuropathy are limited to lifestyle interventions

102. A 48-year-old male with type 1 diabetes takes insulin glargine at bedtime and insulin aspart before each meal. His last A1C was 6.9%. He reports 3 episodes in the past 2 weeks of morning hypoglycemia before eating breakfast (blood glucose levels between 50 mg/dL and 72 mg/dL). Which of the following recommendations is MOST appropriate for this patient?

   A. Decrease breakfast insulin aspart

   B. Decrease lunchtime insulin aspart

   C. Decrease bedtime insulin glargine

   D. Continue current regimen

88

Section 3: Practice Exams

103. Evidence supports which of the following statements about the glycemic index (GI)?

 A. Research studies consistently define a low GI as <55, moderate 56–69, and high >70

 B. Foods with a high glycemic index include ice cream, sugars, and fruit

 C. Swapping low glycemic load foods for higher glycemic load foods may modestly improve glycemia

 D. Foods have similar glycemic effects from one individual to another

104. A 48-year-old patient is newly diagnosed with type 2 diabetes. He has a medical history of myocardial infarction 2 years ago, heart failure (New York Heart Association 3), and hypertension. He works in construction, smokes 1 pack per day, and drinks 2 beers per week. Laboratory values from today are as follows: SCr 0.9 mg/dL, AST 15 mg/dL, ALT 20 mg/dL. Which of the following is the most compelling reason to avoid metformin therapy in this patient?

 A. Alcohol consumption

 B. Hypertension

 C. Renal insufficiency

 D. Heart failure

105. Which of the following is a TRUE statement concerning fructose?

 A. Fructose is a disaccharide found naturally in fruits

 B. Fructose has a greater glycemic effect compared with sucrose

 C. Beverages with high fructose corn syrup should be limited or avoided

 D. People with diabetes should avoid all types of fructose due to the effect on triglycerides

106. A physician decides that her patient would benefit from weight loss. Which of the following would be MOST helpful in promoting weight loss?

 A. Pioglitazone

 B. Exenatide

 C. Nateglinide

 D. Glipizide

107. Which of the following statements about gastroparesis is correct?

 A. Gastrointestinal motility is unaffected by glycemic control

 B. Dietary modifications include frequent, small, high-fat meals

 C. Diagnosis is based on clinical symptoms

 D. Symptoms of gastroparesis include nausea, vomiting, abdominal bloating, and early satiety

Review Guide for the CDE® Exam

108. Which of the following is an example of a resistance exercise?

    A. Cycling

    B. Push-ups

    C. Jogging

    D. Sprinting

109. Which of the following is NOT a concern with pioglitazone?

    A. Weight loss

    B. Bladder cancer

    C. Heart failure exacerbation

    D. Osteoporosis and increased fracture risk

110. Which of the following is TRUE regarding the warm-up phase of an exercise session?

    A. Strong evidence supports stretching prior to an aerobic session to prevent muscle injury

    B. The heart rate should be elevated during the warm-up phase

    C. Stretching for 10–15 minutes prior to an exercise session is recommended to warm up muscles prior to an exercise session

    D. The warm-up phase includes doing an activity at a slower speed or lower intensity for 5–10 minutes

111. A 38-year-old patient with type 2 diabetes presents for follow-up. She takes metformin 1 g with breakfast (8 AM) and dinner (6 PM). She also takes detemir 15 units before breakfast (8 AM) and before bedtime (10 PM). Her average self-monitored blood glucose levels are 136 mg/dL at 8 AM, 132 mg/dL at 6 PM, and 220 mg/dL at 10 PM. Which of the following represents the MOST appropriate change to her regimen?

    A. Increase 8 AM detemir to 20 units

    B. Increase 10 PM detemir to 20 units

    C. Move 6 PM metformin dose to 10 PM

    D. Add predinner (6 PM) aspart

112. Which of the following medications is best to target postprandial blood glucose?

    A. Pioglitazone

    B. Repaglinide

    C. Metformin

    D. Insulin glargine

90

Section 3: Practice Exams

113. You are working in a group practice and a medical intern calls to ask you how to initiate insulin therapy. The patient is 63 years old, weighs 280 lbs, and is 6 feet, 5 inches tall (Note: overweight = BMI 25–29.9; obesity = BMI >30). Which of the following is the MOST appropriate weight-based insulin dose recommendation for this patient according to the current ADA Standards of Care?

    A. Degludec insulin 16 units at bedtime

    B. Regular insulin 10 units at bedtime

    C. Glargine insulin 36 units at bedtime

    D. Detemir insulin 25 units at bedtime

114. Which of the following is the MOST appropriate exercise recommendation for individuals with severe peripheral neuropathy?

    A. Avoid all weight-bearing exercises

    B. Individuals without acute foot ulcers should engage in moderate-intensity walking

    C. Individuals with a foot injury or open sore should avoid non-weight-bearing exercises

    D. Use chair exercises only

115. Oral complications of diabetes include all EXCEPT which of the following?

    A. Periodontitis and tooth loss

    B. Gingivitis

    C. Dental abscesses

    D. Dental caries

116. JB is a 34-year-old female with type 1 diabetes on insulin pump therapy. Her insulin-to-carbohydrate ratio is 1:12. She is about to sit down and eat a dinner that contains 42 grams of carbohydrate, and her sensitivity factor is 58. Her target range is 90 to 120 mg/dL. Her current glucose is 165 mg/dL. Which of the following is the most appropriate bolus dose for this patient?

    A. 3.5 units

    B. 4.0 units

    C. 4.5 units

    D. 5.0 units

117. Which of the following is NOT an effect of GLP-1 mimetic agents such as liraglutide and exenatide?

    A. Promotes satiety in the brain

    B. Increases glucagon secretion from alpha cells

    C. Decreases gastric emptying and motility

    D. Enhances insulin secretion from beta cells

91

Review Guide for the CDE® Exam

118. PB is a 43-year-old male with type 1 diabetes and unstable proliferative retinopathy. What type of exercise would be contraindicated for him?

    A. Swimming laps with lane guards

    B. Stationary cycling

    C. Treadmill walking

    D. Push-ups

119. An obese 65-year-old woman was recently diagnosed with type 2 diabetes. She has a past medical history of hypertension, heart failure (New York Heart Association Class III), and chronic kidney disease. Her exam today reveals the following: A1C 7.5%, serum creatinine 1.6 mg/dL, estimated glomerular filtration rate (eGFR) 34 mL/min, blood pressure 110/70 mmHg. Which of the following would be the best choice to improve her glycemic control?

    A. Canagliflozin

    B. Metformin XR

    C. Sitagliptin

    D. Rosiglitazone

120. Which of the following tests is a risk predictor for chromosomal abnormalities and congenital cardiac defects?

    A. Non-stress test (NST)

    B. Biophysical profile (BPP)

    C. Nuchal translucency (NT)

    D. Fetal kick counts

121. MR is an 87-year-old female with a BMI of 32, osteopenia, and sarcopenia (muscle wasting). Which of the following statements is NOT a valid consideration in determining an appropriate nutrition/lifestyle intervention?

    A. A weight loss plan with a 1,000-calorie deficit along with regular exercise would be appropriate considering her obesity

    B. Calcium and vitamin D supplementation may be necessary to meet the requirements for older adults, as they are often difficult to meet with food alone

    C. A modest reduction in calories with an emphasis on nutrient-dense foods and physical activity may help with weight, bone density, and sarcopenia

    D. Due to her age, MR may need to be encouraged to consume more foods containing high-quality protein due to the contribution of protein undernutrition to sarcopenia and morbidity

Section 3: Practice Exams

122. A 34-year-old woman with gestational diabetes (GDM) was well controlled for 2 months with nutritional interventions. Recently her blood glucose levels started rising and her doctor would like to initiate pharmacotherapy. Which of the following would be the MOST appropriate oral therapy recommendation for this patient?

    A. Canagliflozin

    B. Metformin

    C. Repaglinide

    D. Pioglitazone

123. Development of an educational plan requires ALL but which of the following?

    A. Collaboration among the diabetes educator, the patient, the healthcare team, and the family members (as appropriate)

    B. Input from the referring provider

    C. An individualized plan determined by the diabetes educator following assessment

    D. Selection of specific interventions and goals

124. Which of the following injectable agents would be the safest to prescribe for a woman with gestational diabetes during pregnancy?

    A. Liraglutide

    B. NPH insulin

    C. Glargine insulin

    D. Glulisine insulin

125. You suspect that your 35-year-old patient may be functioning at a low literacy level. To assess her literacy skills, which of the following would be most appropriate?

    A. Ask her if she reads the daily newspaper

    B. Ask her about her educational level

    C. Show her a nutrition label and ask questions that require her to read the label

    D. Give her an article and ask her to read it to you

126. Which of the following antihypertensive agents would be MOST appropriate for a pregnant woman with diabetes and chronic hypertension?

    A. Lisinopril

    B. Valsartan

    C. Fosinopril

    D. Methyldopa

Review Guide for the CDE® Exam

127. Which characteristic distinguishes cystic fibrosis-related diabetes (CFRD) from other forms of diabetes?

    A. Polyuria

    B. Polydipsia

    C. Reduced lung function

    D. Fatigue

128. Which of the following is MOST likely to mask the symptoms of hypoglycemia?

    A. Irbesartan

    B. Amlodipine

    C. Propranolol

    D. Hydrochlorothiazide

Use this scenario to answer the next 2 questions.

BJ is a 36-year-old female recently diagnosed with type 2 diabetes. Her BMI is 33 and her A1C is 8.0%. She takes 10 mg of glipizide XL before breakfast. After reviewing results of her self-monitoring of blood glucose (SMBG), you see that her fasting blood glucose (BG) is still above target, yet she complains of being hungry, weak, and shaky in the afternoon. Her weight has increased 4 lbs in 4 weeks.

129. After reviewing results of her self-monitoring of blood glucose (SMBG), you see that her fasting blood glucose (BG) is still above target, yet she complains of being hungry, weak, and shaky in the afternoon. Her weight has increased 4 pounds in 4 weeks. Which of the following changes would be most appropriate for this patient?

    A. Change glipizide XL to 5 mg twice/day

    B. Discontinue glipizide XL and begin metformin

    C. Switch glipizide to glimeperide

    D. Ask her to eat a snack in the afternoon

130. At BJ's session with the diabetes educator, she learned about basic carbohydrate counting and self-monitoring of blood glucose (SMBG). She has discovered through her SMBG that a lot of fruits, starchy foods, and dairy products raise her postmeal blood glucose (BG) more than if she has only vegetables and meat. She has therefore eliminated fruits, starches, milk, and yogurt from her diet. Based on evidence, what would be the best response to her?

    A. Choosing foods solely on the basis of their effect on blood glucose compromises healthy eating

    B. Any type of eating pattern that lowers postprandial blood glucose is recommended

    C. Taking multiple vitamin and calcium supplements will provide the nutrients missing from a low-carb diet plan

    D. Avoiding carbohydrate foods with a moderate or high glycemic index is recommended to improve glycemia

Section 3: Practice Exams

131. Which of the following forms of contraception is associated with an increased risk for the development of type 2 diabetes among breastfeeding women with a history of gestational diabetes?

    A. Diaphragm

    B. IUD

    C. Combination oral contraceptives

    D. Progestin-only oral contraceptives

132. A patient who recently started an angiotensin-converting enzyme inhibitor (ACEI) presents with several complaints. Which of the following is LEAST likely to warrant a medication change?

    A. Dry hacking cough

    B. Swelling of face and tongue

    C. Potassium rise to 5.8 mg/dL

    D. Serum creatinine rise from 1.2 to 1.6 mg/dL

133. Which of the following suggestions demonstrates the most effective communication between you and your patient?

    A. Check your blood sugar on a regular basis

    B. Get plenty of rest

    C. Eat more fiber

    D. Exercise 3 to 5 days per week for 30 minutes

134. A 42-year-old male with type 2 diabetes presents to the clinic for follow-up on his fasting laboratory values. Total cholesterol is 300 mg/dL, triglyceride 683 mg/dL, HDL cholesterol 35 mg/dL, and LDL cholesterol 130 mg/dL. Which of the following represents the MOST appropriate drug therapy option for this patient?

    A. Atorvastatin 10 mg daily

    B. Pitavastatin 1 mg daily

    C. Fenofibrate 145 mg daily

    D. Ezetimibe 10 mg daily

135. Which of the following statements about sexuality and diabetes is TRUE?

    A. Issues of sexuality, sexual functioning, and reproductive health should only be addressed with adults

    B. Erectile dysfunction occurs in men with diabetes at an earlier age than in the general population

    C. Sexual difficulties are rare in women

    D. This is a sensitive topic and sexual concerns should only be addressed if raised by the patient

SECTION 3: PRACTICE EXAMS

95

Review Guide for the CDE® Exam

136. What does the evidence reveal about the effect of weight loss on glycemia and diabetes prevention?

    A. Improves glycemia in most individuals with diabetes

    B. Does not prevent diabetes unless weight loss is >20%

    C. Improves glycemia more in individuals who are insulin deficient

    D. Has less effect on individuals with long-standing diabetes

137. Which of the following is NOT included in the American Diabetes Association's (ADA's) therapeutic lifestyle change (TLC) recommendations for patients with diabetes and dyslipidemia?

    A. Reduce saturated fat

    B. Reduce dietary cholesterol

    C. Add plant stanols and sterols

    D. Limit amount of dietary fiber

138. The American Diabetes Association (ADA) recommends that bariatric surgery be considered for which of the following?

    A. Children over age 14 with a BMI >35 kg/m^2 and inadequately controlled type 2 diabetes

    B. Adults with a BMI >30 kg/m^2 and inadequately controlled type 2 diabetes

    C. Adults with a BMI >35 kg/m^2 and inadequately controlled type 2 diabetes

    D. Children over age 16 with a BMI >40 kg/m^2 and inadequately controlled type 2 diabetes

139. There is an increased risk of myalgias when simvasta tin is combined with which of the following agents?

    A. Cholestyramine

    B. Ezetimibe

    C. Gemfibrozil

    D. Omega-3 fish oil

140. Higher remission rates following bariatric surgery are associated with which of the following?

    A. Higher BMI

    B. Higher A1C

    C. Shorter duration of type 2 diabetes

    D. Insulin use

Section 3: Practice Exams

141. Current recommendations by the American Diabetes Association (ADA) for exercise in children with diabetes include at least

    A. 30 minutes of a structured exercise session most days.

    B. 60 minutes of moderate-intensity physical activity most days of the week.

    C. 60 minutes of vigorous physical activity every day.

    D. 150 minutes/week of moderate-intensity exercise such as walking.

142. Which of the following is NOT a potential side effect of niacin?

    A. Flushing

    B. Hepatotoxicity

    C. Hyperuricemia

    D. Hypoglycemia

143. Evidence has shown that matching the premeal insulin with the carbohydrate in the meal in individuals with type 1 diabetes can decrease A1C levels by approximately

    A. 0.3%.

    B. 0.5%.

    C. 1.0%.

    D. 2.0%.

144. A 62-year-old man with type 2 diabetes was recently started on niacin. He calls the clinic after 2 days complaining of severe hot flashes and flushing. Which of the following would be the best recommendation for this patient?

    A. Discontinue niacin for 2 weeks, then restart

    B. Take aspirin 325 mg about 30 minutes before niacin

    C. Take a hot shower about 15 minutes after start of flushing

    D. Drink a hot liquid such as tea with the niacin dose

145. According to the American Diabetes Association's (ADA's) Standards of Care, which of the following statements regarding screening for type 2 diabetes in children is correct?

    A. Screening is recommended for children who are overweight and have 2 or more risk factors for diabetes

    B. Screening should begin prior to puberty in high-risk, obese children

    C. Yearly screening is recommended for children deemed to be at high risk

    D. The oral glucose tolerance test (OGTT) is the preferred diagnostic test in individuals under 18 years old

Review Guide for the CDE® Exam

146. For a patient who presents with hypertriglyceridemia (TG >500 mg/dL), which of the following therapeutic options would be MOST appropriate?

    A. Garlic

    B. Fish oil

    C. Ezetimibe

    D. Plant sterols

147. A 52-year-old male patient with hypertension on lisinopril 20 mg and hydrochlorothiazide 12.5 mg daily presents to the clinic for evaluation of his cholesterol. He reports good medication compliance, works out at the YMCA 3 times a week, and follows a low-fat diet. He drinks 1 or 2 beers on the weekend but does not smoke. He states that heart disease "runs in his family" and that his father died of myocardial infarction at age 61. His lipid profile is as follows: total cholesterol 216 mg/dL, triglyceride 200 mg/dL, HDL cholesterol 32 mg/dL. Based on this presentation, how many major risk factors does this patient have?

    A. One

    B. Two

    C. Three

    D. Four

148. Which of the following is NOT a socioeconomic barrier that may impact the physical activity level of adults?

    A. Financial constraints

    B. Unsafe neighborhoods

    C. Proximity or access to gyms

    D. Lack of motivation

149. Patients with peripheral arterial disease (PAD) are considered to have the same atherosclerotic cardiovascular disease (ASCVD) risk as patients with established coronary artery disease (CAD). Which of the following would also classify a patient with ASCVD?

    A. Ankle brachial index greater than 9

    B. Abdominal aortic aneurysm

    C. hs-CRP less than 1 mg/dL

    D. Framingham 10-year risk less than 10%

98

Section 3: Practice Exams

150. According to the American Diabetes Association (ADA), which drug therapy is recommended as the initial agent in patients with type 2 diabetes?

    A. Acarbose

    B. Sulfonylureas

    C. Metformin

    D. SGLT-2 inhibitors

151. Women with gestational diabetes have an increased risk of which of the following?

    A. Offspring with cystic fibrosis

    B. Type 2 diabetes later in life

    C. Obesity

    D. Offspring with heart defects

152. According to the Food and Drug Administration (FDA) guidelines, women should avoid which of the following foods during pregnancy?

    A. Swordfish

    B. Non-organic foods

    C. Raw fruits and vegetables

    D. Salmon

153. A pregnant woman with a past medical history of type 2 diabetes, coronary artery disease (CAD), and hypercholesterolemia uncontrolled by lifestyle presents for evaluation. Which of the following drug therapy options would be the best choice for this patient?

    A. Niacin

    B. Rosuvastatin

    C. Gemfibrozil

    D. Colesevelam

154. MS is a 31-year-old pregnant female with type 2 diabetes. She has a sedentary job as a receptionist. In the absence of medical complications, which is the MOST appropriate physical activity recommendation for MS?

    A. Avoidance of all physical activity

    B. 30 minutes of moderate physical activity most days of the week

    C. Continuing usual activity

    D. Flexibility and upper body exercises only

Review Guide for the CDE® Exam

155. Children with type 1 diabetes who also have celiac disease should be advised to do which of the following?

  A. Avoid foods containing wheat, barley, and rye

  B. Reduce consumption of foods with a high sodium content

  C. Limit foods containing barley, white wheat, and rice

  D. Avoid foods containing rice, corn, and wheat

156. LT is a 48-year-old female with type 1 diabetes of 24-year duration, hypertension, retinopathy, and neuropathy. She is currently on a basal/bolus insulin regimen. In discussing her self-monitoring of blood glucose (SMBG) log, she complains of periodic episodes of hypoglycemia following a meal, even when taking her rapid-acting insulin at the start of the meal. She also complains of poor appetite, nausea, bloating, and diarrhea (sometimes nocturnal), which have increased in frequency over the past 6 months. Which of the following would you suspect to be the MOST likely diagnosis?

  A. Irritable bowel syndrome (IBS)

  B. Gastroparesis

  C. Gastroesophageal reflux disease (GERD)

  D. Gastrointestinal virus

157. Patients with which of the following diabetes complications should avoid vigorous aerobic or resistance exercise?

  A. Proliferative diabetic retinopathy

  B. Gastroparesis

  C. Peripheral neuropathy

  D. Nephropathy

158. A 52-year-old male with type 2 diabetes and high cholesterol presents without complaints to clinic for follow-up. His current medications include metformin 1 g twice daily and rosuvastatin 20 mg daily. His current fasting glucose laboratory values are 260 mg/dL, triglyceride 683 mg/dL, HDL cholesterol 38 mg/dL, and LDL cholesterol 114 mg/dL. Which of the following represents the MOST appropriate drug therapy option for this patient?

  A. Add fish oil

  B. Switch to fluvastatin

  C. Switch to simvastatin

  D. Add colesevelam

Section 3: Practice Exams

159. WP states that he will try to follow the lifestyle changes you suggest because he knows it will improve his blood glucose, but he does NOT know if he can give up his sweets. What stage of behavior change is he exhibiting?

    A. Precontemplation

    B. Contemplation

    C. Preparation

    D. Action

160. ST is a 37-year-old woman with type 2 diabetes. She takes glargine insulin 24 units at bedtime and 8 units of lispro before each meal. Her fasting glucoses range from 52 to 240 mg/dL, 72 to 125 mg/dL before lunch, 85–115 mg/dL before dinner, and 105–140 mg/dL before bed. Her A1C is 7.2% and one glucose at 2:00 AM was 56 mg/dL. Which of the following is the MOST appropriate recommendation?

    A. Reduce lispro at meals

    B. Decrease glargine at bedtime

    C. Increase glargine at bedtime

    D. Increase lispro at meals

161. A 45-year-old female patient is newly diagnosed with type 2 diabetes. Her A1C is 8.8%, her serum creatinine is 0.6%, and her BMI is 22 kg/m^2. Which of the following drug therapy options would be MOST appropriate?

    A. Exenatide

    B. Saxagliptin

    C. Acarbose

    D. Metformin

162. Which of the following medications is MOST associated with weight gain?

    A. Exenatide

    B. Metformin

    C. Acarbose

    D. Nateglinide

163. Which of the following statements about the dawn phenomenon is NOT true?

    A. It is a normal physiologic process

    B. Hormonal basis is thought to be due mainly to overnight growth hormone and cortisol secretion

    C. It is usually recurrent and modestly elevates most morning glucose levels

    D. Insulin pump therapy has not been shown to be effective in controlling the dawn phenomenon

101

Review Guide for the CDE® Exam

164. You are counseling your patient on limiting trans fats and saturated fats to facilitate reduction of LDL cholesterol. Which of the following foods is MOST likely to contain artificial trans fats?

    A. Liquid margarine

    B. Avocado

    C. Biscuits

    D. Soybean oil

165. Which of the following agents is LEAST likely to cause hypoglycemia in an active adult?

    A. Glyburide

    B. Sitagliptin

    C. Repaglinide

    D. Regular insulin

166. RW tells you she is following a vegan-style eating plan. Which of the following foods would be included in her eating plan?

    A. Spinach, eggs, and milk

    B. Fish, brown rice, and sweet potatoes

    C. Yogurt, carrots, and barley

    D. Lentils, black beans, and broccoli

167. A 43-year-old African American female patient with type 2 diabetes for 8 years and hypothyroidism for 10 years presents to the clinic complaining of a toothache. Her current medications include levothyroxine 0.75 mcg daily, metformin 1 g twice daily, and glipizide 10 mg twice daily. Her laboratory values today are as follows: A1C 7.2%, fasting plasma glucose 268 mg/dL, TSH 0.8 uIU/mL. Which of the following is the MOST likely reason why her fasting plasma glucose is elevated today?

    A. Hyperthyroidism

    B. Secondary glipizide failure

    C. Secondary infection of tooth

    D. Progressive beta-cell destruction

168. You encourage your patients to consume more whole grains as recommended by the American Diabetes Association (ADA) and the US Dietary Guidelines. Which of the following are considered whole grains?

    A. Quinoa, brown rice, and long-grain white rice

    B. Oatmeal, quinoa, and whole wheat flour

    C. Honey wheat flour, jasmine rice, and flour tortillas

    D. Millet, white wheat flour, and corn

Section 3: Practice Exams

169. A 54-year-old male with type 2 diabetes presents for follow-up on maximum dose metformin. He wants to lose weight but is also concerned about hypoglycemia. His A1C is 7.8% and his serum creatinine is 0.8%. Which of the following drug therapy options would be MOST appropriate?

    A. Sitagliptin

    B. Canagliflozin

    C. Glargine insulin

    D. Glulisine insulin

170. A patient with an irregular meal schedule presents to the clinic for follow-up. He takes metformin 1 g twice daily and his current A1C is 7.4%. He reports drinking coffee for breakfast, eating crackers for lunch, and eating a large evening meal when he comes home from work. Review of his self-monitored blood glucose records reveals elevated values after his large evening meal. Which of the following would be the best option to improve his glycemic control?

    A. Increase metformin

    B. Add glargine insulin

    C. Add nateglinide

    D. Add glyburide

171. MT is on a basal/bolus regimen of 32 units of glargine every night at bedtime and 8 units of lispro before each meal. Based on the following self-monitored blood glucose pattern, which of the following is the most appropriate recommendation?

Breakfast	Lunch	Dinner	Bedtime
75	115	103	110
98	167	96	97
86	152	94	102
102	148	87	115

    A. Increase the bedtime glargine

    B. Increase prebreakfast lispro

    C. Increase prebreakfast and predinner lispro

    D. Decrease bedtime glargine

103

Review Guide for the CDE® Exam

172. RJ, a 24-year-old male with type 1 diabetes, is on a basal/bolus regimen of twice-daily detemir and aspart before meals and large snacks. He is experiencing nausea and vomiting and has a slightly elevated fever. His glucose that morning was 243 mg/dL and his urine is positive for trace ketones. Which of the following is the best advice for this patient?

    A. Limit carbohydrate intake

    B. Stop and/or hold basal insulin until symptoms subside

    C. Limit fluid intake to 2 oz per hour

    D. Continue to test blood glucoses 4 times a day

173. "I have looked at all the diets out there. I think I'll stick with the meal plan I learned about at my last diabetes clinic visit." This statement indicates the individual is in what stage of change?

    A. Precontemplation

    B. Contemplation

    C. Preparation

    D. Maintenance

174. Which of the following classes of medications is associated with fluid retention and edema?

    A. Biguanides

    B. Thiazolidinediones

    C. DPP-4 inhibitors

    D. SGLT-2 inhibitors

175. Which of the following statements about the 1,5-Anhydroglucitrol (1,5-AG) Blood Test (GlycoMark®) is correct?

    A. Provides insight about short-term glycemic control as well as glycemic excursions

    B. Is especially useful in patients with an A1C that exceeds 8%

    C. During times of hyperglycemia, reabsorption of 1,5-AG is increased

    D. Can be used in patients with advanced kidney and liver disease

176. The American Diabetes Association's (ADA's) Standards of Care for the use of aspirin (acetyl-salicylic acid or ASA) therapy include ALL but which of the following? Aspirin can be used as a

    A. secondary prevention in those who have a history of cardiovascular disease.

    B. primary prevention in men aged >50 and at least 1 major cardiovascular (CVD) risk factor.

    C. primary prevention in women aged >60 with at least 1 major cardiovascular CVD risk factor.

    D. primary prevention in adults of any age with retinopathy.

104

Section 3: Practice Exams

177. Which of the following cholesterol-lowering drugs can be used safely in pregnancy?

    A. Fenofibrate

    B. Atorvastatin

    C. Colesevelam

    D. Evolocumab

178. Which of the following statements about blood glucose goals for critically ill patients is TRUE?

    A. Insulin therapy should be initiated for the treatment of persistent hyperglycemia starting at a threshold of no greater than 180 mg/dL and then maintained in a range of 140 to 180 mg/dL

    B. Insulin therapy should be initiated for the treatment of persistent hyperglycemia starting at a threshold of no greater than 240 mg/dL and then maintained in a range of 140 to 180 mg/dL

    C. Insulin therapy should be initiated for the treatment of persistent hyperglycemia starting at a threshold of no greater than 180 mg/dL and then maintained in a range of 110 to 140 mg/dL

    D. Insulin therapy should be initiated for the treatment of persistent hyperglycemia starting at a threshold of no greater than 150 mg/dL and then maintained in a range of 110 to 140 mg/dL

179. Which of the following is NOT a risk factor for hypoglycemia in patients with type 2 diabetes?

    A. Delayed or skipped meal

    B. Alcohol consumption without food intake

    C. Significantly increased physical activity

    D. Weight gain

180. Which of the following statements regarding smoking and diabetes is NOT correct?

    A. Smoking is related to the earlier development of microvascular complications

    B. Smoking is associated with an increased risk of premature death

    C. Tobacco use is associated with increased progression of peripheral artery disease (PAD) and increased risk of amputation

    D. Smoking cessation programs have been shown to be less effective for individuals with diabetes than in the general population

181. Intensive glucose control among patients with type 2 diabetes is associated with which of the following?

    A. Weight loss

    B. Elevations in triglycerides

    C. Decreased cardiovascular mortality

    D. Decreased progression of retinopathy

SECTION 3:
PRACTICE EXAMS

105

Review Guide for the CDE® Exam

182. Insulin requirements during pregnancy
    A. are lower in women with >150% of desirable body weight.
    B. increase dramatically after delivery.
    C. increase progressively throughout gestation.
    D. are increased during the first trimester of pregnancy.

183. Management of hypoglycemia unawareness and unresponsiveness includes ALL but which of the following?
    A. Reduced goals for glucose and A1C levels
    B. Increased size of mealtime boluses
    C. Avoidance of hypoglycemia
    D. Blood glucose management training

184. Which of the following agents is NOT recommended for women who are breastfeeding?
    A. Glipizide
    B. Metformin
    C. Acarbose
    D. Sitagliptin

185. Diabetes-related distress
    A. has little impact on metabolic control.
    B. is rarely severe enough to require referral to a mental health professional.
    C. is less common than depression among people with diabetes.
    D. is responsive to interventions, including DSMES.

186. Which of the following statements regarding insulin storage is TRUE?
    A. Storage guidelines for used or unused insulin vials and insulin cartridges and disposable prefilled pens are the same
    B. Unopened, but not opened vials of insulin may be stored at room temperature for 1 month
    C. Unopened refrigerated insulin vials and pens can be used up to 1 month past their expiration date
    D. Storage guidelines for used or unused insulin cartridges and disposable prefilled pens differ based on the type of insulin they contain

106

Section 3: Practice Exams

187. RT is admitted to your inpatient Medical Surgical unit. During your assessment, you note that according to his admission labs his A1C is 6.8% but glucoses since admission have all been greater than 250 mg/dL. Which of the following is the best explanation for the disparity between A1C and point-of-care glucose values?

A. Uncontrolled diabetes for several months

B. Recent improvement of his glycemic control

C. Recent insulin dose increase

D. Controlled diabetes with recent physiologic stress

188. Which of the following statements regarding program accreditation and recognition is TRUE?

A. At least 1 CDE must be on staff for a program to be accredited

B. Accreditation or recognition automatically guarantees reimbursement

C. Programs must assess and document the diabetes self-management, education, and support needs of each participant

D. The diabetes education program must be 10 hours in length

189. Which of the following Food and Drug Administration (FDA) categories of glucose-lowering medications in pregnancy indicates that the product is contraindicated in women who are or may become pregnant?

A. Categories A and B

B. Category C

C. Category D

D. Category X

190. You are seeing RZ, a 50-year-old man (BMI 38 kg/m²) with type 2 diabetes, for nutrition and weight loss counseling. He is currently receiving NPH and regular insulin twice a day before breakfast and his evening meal. He complains of frequent middle-of-the-night hypoglycemia and elevated fasting blood glucose levels. You would

A. reduce his NPH before dinner.

B. reduce both his regular and NPH before dinner.

C. increase his bedtime snack.

D. move his NPH insulin dose to bedtime.

191. Which of the following statements regarding type 2 diabetes in older adults is NOT correct?

A. Diagnostic criteria are less stringent for older adults

B. The risk of hypoglycemia is increased among older adults

C. Older adults rarely present with the symptoms of hyperglycemia

D. Physical limitations and alterations in daily activities are more common among older adults with diabetes than those without

Review Guide for the CDE® Exam

192. A simple tool used in motivational interviewing is the acronym DARN, which stands for

    A. denial, activities, reasons, and need.

    B. desire, ability, reasons, and need.

    C. desire, ability, rapport, and nature.

    D. denial, activities, reasons, and need.

193. Which of the following topics is best handled by problem solving versus direct instruction?

    A. Symptoms of hypoglycemia and hyperglycemia

    B. Measuring blood glucose and/or ketone levels

    C. Sick-day rules

    D. Strategies to resolve barriers to maintenance of self-management behaviors

194. You are seeing SM, a 30-year-old pregnant female with type 2 diabetes at 20 weeks' gestation. She has just gone to the lab to have her A1C level drawn and questions you regarding recommended target range to minimize risks for her baby. Which of the following is the most appropriate A1C target during the second trimester of pregnancy?

    A. <6.0%

    B. <6.3%

    C. <6.5%

    D. <7.0%

195. Which of the following statements regarding chronic kidney disease (CKD) is NOT true?

    A. Protein intake should be limited to 0.8 g/kg per day

    B. Patients with CKD have an elevated risk for cardiovascular disease

    C. Optimizing blood glucose and blood pressure control has not been shown to delay progression

    D. Incretin mimetics are not recommended for patients with a glomerular filtration rate (GFR) <60 ml/min/1.73m^2

196. Diabetes self-management and support has been shown to improve A1C by as much as _____% in people with type 2 diabetes.

    A. 0.5

    B. 0.8

    C. 1.0

    D. 1.3

Section 3: Practice Exams

Use the following scenario to answer the next 4 questions.

Your hospitalized patient is being transitioned from an intravenous (IV) drip to subcutaneous insulin injections. You must calculate the subcutaneous dose for your patient, who received 5 units of rapid-acting insulin per hour over the previous 24 hours.

197. Calculate his total daily dose.
    A. 120 units
    B. 96 units
    C. 80 units
    D. 64 units

198. Calculate his basal dose.
    A. 40 units
    B. 48 units
    C. 60 units
    D. 100 units

199. The patient will be started on a carbohydrate-controlled diet for dinner. Calculate his bolus dose.
    A. 5 units
    B. 10 units
    C. 15 units
    D. 16 units

200. When should the first dose of subcutaneous insulin be administered?
    A. Two hours before the insulin drip is discontinued
    B. Four hours before the insulin drip is discontinued
    C. Immediately following discontinuation of the drip
    D. At bedtime on the day the drip is discontinued

SECTION

4

Answer Key

**In the answer rationales below, a capital A, B, C, or D
within parentheses references answer choices.**

Section 2: Self-Assessment Tests

Assessment of Diabetes and Prediabetes

1. **A.** Initial teaching should focus on survival level skills that the newly diagnosed patient would need to safely manage her disease upon discharge, ie, the signs and symptoms as well as the appropriate treatment of hypoglycemia. Information on the epidemiology of diabetes (B), the association between hyperglycemia and defects (C), and carbohydrate counting (D), although important, is not information/skills that are needed immediately.

2. **B.** Diabetes education should be tailored to patient preferences with regard to timing, delivery method, and use of technology. This young patient is very comfortable with technology and is likely very busy based on the number of interruptions during the session. Scheduling education sessions in the morning (A) may be convenient for the educator but not the patient. Text messaging and constant contact with friends are considered appropriate for young patients, so educators should not expect patients to leave their cell phones at home (C). Social networking with peers is important for patients; however, young patients often prefer online networking forums over face-to-face meetings (D).

3. **D.** Many adults who are illiterate are able to successfully hide their literacy deficit. The other three choices (A, B, and C) are all commonly held misconceptions regarding low literacy and are not accurate.

111

Review Guide for the CDE® Exam

4. **C.**   His medications are not likely to be the cause of his inability to lose weight. It is likely his food choices that are the problem, particularly since he has to eat on the road and, as a result, can face more challenges selecting healthy food choices. Assessing eating habits is one key component of a diabetes assessment. Answer A is incorrect because it doesn't address the root problem—weight gain. Furthermore, glucose tablet use is not likely to contribute to weight management issues. Metformin typically does not cause weight gain, but rather a 2–5 kg weight loss (B). Answer D is incorrect because the question is irrelevant to the problem and unrelated to weight management.

5. **C.**   It is recommended that a foot examination be performed at every diabetes care visit. Although a dilated eye examination (A) and gastric emptying test (D) are diabetes specific assessments, both require referral to a specialist. A tuberculin skin test is not diabetes specific (B).

6. **B.**   The BMI for normal weight is 18.5–24.9. A BMI of <18.5 is underweight (A). A BMI of 25–29.9 is overweight (C). A BMI of 30 or greater is obese (D).

7. **A.**   An intense fear of gaining weight or becoming fat, even though underweight, is the classic description of anorexia nervosa. Bulimia nervosa is characterized by recurrent episodes of binge eating often followed by inappropriate compensatory behavior (such as self-induced vomiting, misuse of laxatives, diuretics, or enemas, or excessive exercise) to prevent weight gain (B). Binge-eating disorder is characterized by repeated episodes of binge eating, but in the absence of compensatory behaviors to prevent weight gain. It's often accompanied by marked stress about the binge eating (C). Purging is one characteristic of bulimia nervosa. It is inappropriate compensatory behavior (such as self-induced vomiting, misuse of laxatives, diuretics, or enemas, or excessive exercise) to prevent weight gain (D).

8. **C.**   Individuals with type 2 diabetes are generally ketone resistant. Individuals in DKA are also dehydrated (B) and hyperglycemic (A). Neurologic changes (lethargy and mild confusion) are less common in DKA (D) but can occur.

9. **B.**   Since A1C is based on normal hemoglobin, hemoglobinopathies can affect the test in three ways: 1) Altering the normal process of glycation from HbA to A1C; 2) Causing an abnormal peak on chromatography making the estimation or A1C unreliable; 3) Making the red blood cells more prone to hemolysis, thereby decreasing the time for glycosylation to occur and thereby producing a falsely low A1C. There is a lack of evidence to support interference of low-dose aspirin usage with A1C result. Ingesting large doses of aspirin may, however, impact A1C result (A). White blood cell count is not related to hemoglobin A1C, which is a measure of the amount of glucose attached to the hemoglobin in the red blood cells (C). Oral contraceptives do not affect the accuracy of A1C result (D).

Section 4: Answer Key

10. **B.** Remind him that it can take up to 12 weeks to see an effect with a TZD. Thiazoli-dinediones improve glycemic control by up-regulating genes that encode for glucose transporter formation and promoting fat mobilization from visceral stores to deposit in subcutaneous cells. In some patients, improvement in glycemic control from these mechanisms may not be observed for 8 to 12 weeks. This patient already follows a prescribed diet and exercise program, so it is not appropriate to further intensify these lifestyle interventions (A and D). Once the TZD is given enough time to work, this patient may be referred back to his primary care physician for additional interventions (C).

11. **B.** Drug-induced nausea is common with pramlintide, occurring in up to 48% of patients, making B the correct answer. Gradual titration to the recommended dose reduces this reaction.

12. **D.** The discrepancy could likely be related to the patient's SMBG technique. The inconsistency lies between the A1C of 11% (estimated average glucose of 310 mg/dL) and the 14-day meter average of 130 mg/dL. In prioritizing the course of action to determine the cause for the discrepancy, having the patient demonstrate his monitoring technique is a simple first step with no associated additional cost. If this doesn't resolve the issue, further action can be taken. A random, non-fasting plasma glucose will not provide any valuable information in this scenario (A). While iron-deficiency anemia can affect A1C results, anemia wouldn't be the likely cause since both the A1C and the fasting lab sample were markedly higher than the patient's results and it's unlikely the patient developed anemia within the previous two weeks (B). Falsifying records would not be a likely cause from a pastor (C), but could be considered.

13. **A.** Drawing up an accurate insulin dose and injecting it correctly requires both dexterity and visual acuity. These are key areas to assess when initiating insulin therapy. Balance does not typically impact ability to use vial and syringe (B). Hearing does not impact insulin injection technique (C). Visual acuity can impact ability to draw up an accurate insulin dose and inject it correctly; hearing does not impact insulin injection technique (D).

14. **B.** Expenses are often a major concern for the elderly. Diminished taste (A) is unrelated to insulin therapy, and altered pain perception (C) is generally not a concern because of the size of the needles currently used. Although physical activity (D) can affect insulin requirements it is generally not a barrier to insulin therapy.

15. **C.** An assessment is necessary for any patient presenting for diabetes education. Even though the person described in the question is a healthcare professional, this does not mean that the diabetes educator should skip the assessment and move on to providing specific information about the disease or treatment options (A, B, D).

113

Review Guide for the CDE® Exam

Interventions for Diabetes and Prediabetes

1. **B.** Role-playing is the most appropriate intervention because it can help the patient practice, express, explore, discuss, and share information. The patient voices understanding of meal planning concepts; however, this form of active learning can facilitate sharing of additional information and allow her to practice.

   There are no clues in the question indicating that social anxiety is the root of the problem (A). Answer C is incorrect because this action does not address the root of the problem—what she orders when eating out. Answer D is incorrect because she already voices understanding of this information.

2. **C.** Active learning is more effective with children. Printed material (A), slide presentation (B), and live lecture (D) are all forms of passive learning and therefore incorrect.

3. **C.** Self-behavior skills such as self-monitoring of blood glucose or insulin injection technique are best taught by demonstration with direct observation of return demonstration. Overview lectures, print materials, and role-playing scenarios (A, B, and D) may supplement skill demonstration but should not replace it.

4. **D.** The current guidelines recommend 15–20 grams of carbohydrate, preferably glucose, to treat a hypoglycemic episode. Carbohydrate sources high in protein are not recommended to treat or prevent hypoglycemia in persons with type 2 diabetes as protein appears to increase insulin response without increasing plasma glucose. A, B, and C all contain protein.

5. **B.** Patients with diabetes are free to operate private vehicles, but should be advised to take appropriate precautions (A). Patients should not blindly consume carbohydrates (C) or be restricted to unrealistic testing regimens (D).

6. **C.** Fructosamine, a glycated serum protein test, measures glycemic control over the previous 2–3 weeks. Fructosamine values are particularly useful in evaluation of recent glycemic control in gestational diabetes.

   Answer A is incorrect because it reflects average blood glucose levels for approximately the previous 3 months. A1C would not offer valuable insight on recent blood glucose control.

   Monitoring urinary ketones in women with gestational diabetes is used to detect inadequate food intake (starvation ketosis) and provide warning of impending metabolic decompensation, not to reflect recent blood glucose control (B).

   Microalbumin testing evaluates the advancement of diabetic kidney disease. The presence of microalbuminuria represents an early phase of nephropathy (D).

SECTION 4: ANSWER KEY

Section 4: Answer Key

7. **D.** The *ADA Standards of Medical Care in Diabetes* recommend an A1C goal of <7.5% as the target for children of all age groups (D). A lower goal (<7%) is reasonable if it can be achieved without excessive hypoglycemia. Previous recommendations suggested higher goals for young patients due to concerns about cognitive impairment, but these issues have not been substantiated by current data.

8. **A.** Weight loss of 10 kg or 20 lbs. can be expected to reduce systolic blood pressure (SBP) by 5 to 20 mm Hg. Restricting salt intake (B) to 2.4 g per day or alcohol intake (D) to fewer than 2 drinks per day only reduces SBP by 2 to 8 mm Hg and 2 to 4 mm Hg respectively. Aerobic exercise (C) 30 minutes daily reduces SBP by 4–9 mm Hg.

9. **D.** Alcohol can enhance glucose-stimulated insulin secretion and reduce gluconeogenesis (making B incorrect) in the liver, leading to an increased risk of hypoglycemia in individuals taking insulin or insulin secretagogues especially if food intake has been restricted.

10. **A.** Given the patient's age and history of peripheral artery disease, a graded exercise test would give key information on how his heart responds to exertion—information he must know before beginning an exercise program in the absence of exercise over the last 10 years. Otherwise, he may put himself at undue risk for a cardiac event. The presence of atherosclerosis in the leg arteries is a strong indicator that there may also be atherosclerosis in the arteries of the heart.

    Answers B, C, and D are incorrect because they do not address the primary concern, which is his cardiac health and preventing a cardiac event. Pain at rest would definitely not signify improvement (he should not experience pain at rest) (D).

11. **A.** Exercise improves insulin sensitivity, increases HDL, and improves strength and physical work capacity. It also reduces plasma triglycerides and cholesterol levels and enhances fibrolysis, making A the only correct choice.

12. **B.** The essential education points for a patient new to insulin include dose preparation (C), safe needle disposal (D), and insulin storage (A). It is important to prioritize education goals so that the patient does not become overwhelmed with information. Insulin adjustment for sick days (B) can be addressed in a follow-up visit.

13. **B.** Metformin is generally weight neutral, and in fact many appreciate a 2–5 kg weight loss. As a monotherapy, metformin does not typically cause hypoglycemia.

    Sulfonylureas typically DO cause weight gain and hypoglycemia (A). TZDs in fact ARE expensive and DO frequently cause weight gain (C). Repaglinide requires 3 times a day dosing and DOES carry an increased risk for hypoglycemia (D).

14. **B.** The patient's triglycerides are below the recommended target of 150 mg/dL (B). His LDL cholesterol is above the recommended target of 100 mg/dL (C) and his total cholesterol is greater than 200 mg/dL (A). His HDL is less than the recommended target of 40 mg/dL (D).

Review Guide for the CDE® Exam

15. **A.** All insulin types are concentrated 100 units per 1 mL except regular U500 insulin, which is 5 times more concentrated (B). Other insulin types should not be mixed with glargine because of irregular disruption of the absorption kinetics of both products (C). Glargine and other insulin products can be administered at the same time, but should be injected in separate areas on the body using different syringes (D).

16. **A.** Continuous quality improvement is a management approach that attempts to correct program shortcomings via program evaluation (B). Outcomes monitoring is the frequency and interval of measuring specific indicators (C). Outcomes measurement is the process of consistently measuring specific indicators (D).

17. **A.** Individuals who have increased visceral fat, which refers to fat deposited around abdominal organs, appear to have a greater risk of type 2 diabetes than those with subcutaneous fat. Intra-abdominal obesity has a greater supply of capillaries, making it more metabolically active than subcutaneous fat or fat on the hips and thighs. As a result, there is a greater flux or turnover of free fatty acids (FFA). In the liver, the FFA contributes to insulin resistance (lipotoxicity). Since FFA may be used as a fuel source instead of glucose, they can contribute to hyperglycemia.

18. **D.** The calculation is as follows: Prebreakfast blood glucose (205 mg/dL) minus his target blood glucose (100 mg/dL) equals 105 mg/dL. Multiply the difference (105 mg/dL) by his correction factor (1 unit per 50 mg/dL) to equal 2 units. Multiply his calculated breakfast carbohydrate intake (50 g) by his insulin-to-carbohydrate ratio (1 unit per 12 g of carbohydrate) to equal 4 units. Add the amount of correction insulin (2 units) to the amount of insulin to compensate for the meal (4 units) to equal 6 units of aspart insulin before breakfast.

19. **C.** It is not the role of the diabetes educator to diagnose and treat eating disorders. However, the educator should be familiar with the clinical features of each type of eating disorder. Excessive exercise, falling weight, and rising blood glucose are suggestive of a possible eating disorder, which may involve intentional insulin omission for weight control purposes.

    A snack before exercising does not address the issue of poor glycemic control. It would provide a few extra calories, but the weight loss, below-normal BMI, and poor glycemic control suggest a possible eating disorder and/or withholding of insulin (A). Physical activity typically reduces basal insulin needs (D). Answer B is incorrect primarily because during the honeymoon, hypoglycemia with subsequent reduced insulin needs is characteristic, not elevated blood glucose.

20. **B.** Corns, calluses, and reddened areas should be treated by a physician/podiatrist. Over-the-counter remedies can cause tissue damage especially in the presence of neuropathy (A). Patients with diabetes should never use sharp instruments on their feet (C); calluses should be treated by a podiatrist. Alcohol should be avoided as it dries the skin (D).

Section 4: Answer Key

21. **B.** NPH insulin 25 units at bedtime is correct. The calculation is as follows: The basal insulin protocol suggests 0.25 units/kg multiplied by the patient's weight (220 lbs divided by 2.2 lbs/kg to equal 100 kg) to equal 25 units (A, B, and C). Answer D is incorrect because glulisine has a short duration of action and would not last through the night.

22. **B.** Fuel homeostasis has 5 phases. In the postabsorptive state, Phase II, plasma insulin levels decrease and glucagon levels begin to rise. Answer D describes Phase V, the secondary prolonged starvation state (24 to 40 days after food consumption). Answer A describes Phase I, the fed state (0 to 3.9 hours after eating), and Answer C describes Phase III, the early starvation state (16 to 47.9 hours after food consumption).

23. **A.** Based on the American Diabetes Association's Standards of Care, while blood pressure and weight should be checked at each diabetes visit, a fasting lipid profile is recommended at diagnosis, initial medical evaluation, and/or at age 40 years and periodically thereafter (B). A1C needs to be checked every 2–3 months (C). A dilated eye exam is recommended annually, in the absence of complications requiring more frequent monitoring (D).

24. **C.** A smoking cessation program since smoking is the most important modifiable cause of premature death for individuals with diabetes, particularly in a man with coronary artery disease, hypertension, and a previous stroke. Although this man may benefit from meeting with a registered dietitian, nothing in the scenario suggests that weight or nutrition is a problem (A and B). There is no evidence of renal impairment presented (D).

25. **C.** Since this patient already has a basic understanding of the effect of carbohydrate on blood glucose and often reads food labels, she could improve her blood glucose control and better manage her weight, while maintaining flexibility in food choices, through implementation of carbohydrate counting with individualized carbohydrate goals. This approach allows for teaching adjustment of the short-acting insulin dose based on carbohydrate intake.

    While a 1,200-calorie exchange plan could help this patient achieve weight loss and tighter blood glucose control, as a first step approach to medical nutrition therapy, the exchange plan would likely be too intensive and restrictive for this patient—her time is crunched, she's feeding a young family, and she is not currently following any type of meal plan (A).

    While MyPlate does provide a basic overview of the components of a nutritionally balanced diet, it does not address the glycemic effect of foods (specifically carbohydrate) (B).

    Glycemic index of foods may be used as a tool to assist in fine-tuning blood glucose control; however, attempting to use glycemic index alone as a meal planning approach is not practical. Glycemic index of a food is affected by many factors (D).

117

Review Guide for the CDE® Exam

26. **D.** This patient is above her A1C goal of less than 7% and requires a change in her regimen (A). Replacing regular insulin with glipizide (B) is unlikely to improve her glycemic control because her pancreas is already unable to produce enough insulin to meet her daily requirements. Likewise, replacing glargine insulin with pioglitazone (C) is unlikely to meet her A1C goal because thiazolidinediones only improve A1C by about 1% when added to insulin. On her current regimen this patient complains of late-onset hypoglycemia following her morning dose of regular insulin. Switching to rapid-acting aspart insulin will provide mealtime coverage without hypoglycemia.

27. **D.** Since our female patient is ready to make changes it will be important to evaluate all self-care behaviors, including blood glucose, food, activity, and medication logs.

28. **C.** Since JL is experiencing nausea and vomiting, glucose tablets, gels, or hard candies are the most easily digested. Juice (A) and regular soda (B) can be used to treat hypoglycemia but would be more likely to accentuate the nausea. Peanut butter crackers are not a good choice to treat hypoglycemia as food high in fat content slows gastric emptying and absorption (D).

29. **C.** Small, frequent meals lead to lessened bloating, lessened early satiety, and lessened possibility of impaired nutritional status. Reduced fat intake may produce less delay in gastric emptying. Reduced fiber intake may decrease the possibility of bezoar formation. Soft foods are more easily digested.

    Answer A is incorrect for the reasons above. Fiber intake should be decreased, rather than increased, to decrease possibility of bezoar formation (B). There is no evidence to support reduced carbohydrate or increased fluid needs beyond JL's typical targets (D).

30. **B.** Physical activity increases hepatic glucose production and increases the glucose supply available in the blood. Insulin decreases (A), epinephrine and norepinephrine both increase (C), and growth hormone and cortisol increase (D).

Disease Management

1. **A.** Choosing the appropriate method of instruction is a critical determinant to effective education. Teaching and learning can occur effectively remotely via computer. Since the student is unavailable during the day, she could e-mail her food records with carb counts to the educator for evaluation and the educator could then respond via e-mail. The method and message must match learner readiness.

    It is not likely that a college student, who typically stays up late, would get up early and be at a 6 AM appointment (B). The student is not likely to choose this option as she wouldn't want to be bothered during the day and draw attention to herself in front of her peers (C). It is not likely that a college student would meet the educator at a restaurant on a Saturday evening, since that typically is the night to socialize with friends (D).

Section 4: Answer Key

2. **C.** It is important for skill mastery that the patient actually perform the skill, thereby making B and D incorrect. A is incorrect because improper cleansing increases the risk of transmitting blood-borne pathogens from one patient to another.

3. **B.** Initiation and maintenance of physical activity can be directly influenced by the education program. Amputation rates, change in blood pressure, and average A1C all depend on the degree of successful achievement of therapeutic goals outside the reach of diabetes self-management education (A, C, and D).

4. **D.** An opportunity for program improvement has been noted, and therefore doing nothing (A) is an incorrect answer. Making a change in format (C) and increasing advertising (B) without first determining the reason for the decline in referrals are also incorrect. Collecting data (provider survey) to better understand (D) the problem is the best response.

5. **B.** Standard 6 of the National Standards for Diabetes Education states that the assessed needs of the individual with prediabetes and diabetes will determine which of the 9 content areas described in Standard 6 should be covered.

6. **C.** The empowerment approach expects the patient to be active in the management of their diabetes, to be provided with the information needed to make informed daily care decisions, and to be responsible for making those decisions. In contrast, the compliance-based approach views the healthcare professional as the expert (A) and utilizes directive instructions (B). Behavioral capacity and expectations are constructs of social cognitive theory (D).

7. **B.** Some patients experience mood changes in response to hypoglycemia; however, this patient reports the same feelings in response to schedule changes. Improving this patient's problem-solving skills (D) might help him to better identify the causes of his feelings but would not identify possible solutions. Nutrition counseling (A) and self-management training (C) would also be unlikely to resolve all causes of his feelings.

8. **B.** Developing relationships with state legislators is very important for diabetes educators in order to promote positive changes in public policy. Exchange networks (A), hospital quality improvement teams (C), and community health screenings (D) improve care for patients with diabetes but do not directly affect public policy.

9. **C.** Outcomes monitoring is the frequency and interval of measuring specific indicators. How outcomes are used for educational and clinical decision making is outcomes management (A). The process of consistently measuring specific indicators is outcomes measurement (B). The result from multiple variables over an extended time is a long-term outcome (D).

119

Review Guide for the CDE® Exam

10. **D.** Improving patient medication compliance as monitored by refill history is an outcome measure that can be directly related to education received during the program. Continuing to provide education through newsletters is important, but just sending out information does not mean that patients apply it to their daily lives (A). Education programs should strive to provide high-quality education that is valued by participants, but satisfaction surveys are mainly useful to evaluate the delivery method (B). Wearing a medical alert bracelet is important for patients with diabetes; however, it does not keep them from being admitted to the emergency room (C).

Section 3: Practice Exams

Exam 1

1. **B.** Place flyers in every prescription bag is correct. In a fee-for-service environment, where patients pay out-of-pocket, the most efficient advertising needs to be directly to the consumer. A regional newspaper (A) is restricted by whether the target population receives the paper. Advertising to local hospital administrators (C) will only reach those patients who were hospitalized, if the hospital administrator chooses to pass on the information. Contacting the top 3 insurance companies (D) would be effective in a managed care environment, but not in this situation.

2. **B.** Sitagliptin 100 mg daily is correct. This patient requires an A1C lowering effect of 1% to 1.5%, which is within the ability of sitagliptin. Because this patient is very active, the risk of hypoglycemia is high and would be increased after adding glipizide (A). Although adding basal insulin (glargine) would be a first tier option according to the American Diabetes Association's (ADA's) guidelines, the listed starting dose is too high, especially considering his current fasting plasma glucose (C). Adding pioglitazone (D) would improve glycemic control; however, it is not appropriate in this patient with a history of bladder cancer. In December 2016, the FDA updated package labeling for pioglitazone to reflect data from additional studies suggesting a link with bladder cancer.

3. **D.** Add ezetimibe 10 mg daily is correct. This patient is appropriately treated with a high intensity statin based on ADA guidelines; however, his response to drug therapy is poor. The 2016 American College of Cardiology (ACC) non-statin guidelines are a companion document to the 2013 ACC recommendations. The non-statin guidelines identify thresholds of >50% reduction of LDL-C from baseline, or LDL <70 mg/dL or non-HDL C <100 mg/dL for this patient with ASCVD and diabetes. Doubling the dose of rosuvastatin (A) will only achieve an additional LDL reduction of 6%, which will not get the patient to goal. Fluvastatin (C) is a less potent statin, so switching also will not achieve this patient's LDL goal. Fish oil (B) affects triglycerides but not LDL-C.

Section 4: Answer Key

4. **C.** Current American Diabetes Association guidelines discourage use of niacin due to efficacy and the increased risk of stroke. Niacin increases free fatty acid flux, which may worsen insulin resistance in patients with diabetes (A). Gemfibrozil inhibits glucuronidation of statins, resulting in statin accumulation and an increased risk of rhabdomyolysis (B). Sustained release niacin from health food stores is associated with increased risk of hepatotoxicity and should be avoided (D).

5. **B.** Continue metformin 1 g twice daily and add glargine insulin at bedtime is correct. The A1C goal of therapy for this patient is less than 7% per the American Diabetes Association's (ADA's) guidelines. Because this patient is above his A1C goal, intensification of therapy is necessary (D). Metformin continues to be effective throughout the lifetime of the patient with type 2 diabetes and should be retained in the absence of contraindications (A). The optimal dose of metformin is 1,000 mg twice daily, so decreasing the dose is inappropriate in this patient (C).

6. **B.** Start irbesartan 150 mg daily is correct. The blood pressure goal for this patient is less than 130/80 mm Hg (D) due to his ASCVD risk, per the ADA guidelines. Diabetes is a compelling indication to use angiotensin-converting enzyme (ACE) inhibitors or angiotensin receptor blockers (ARBs) as first line agents to achieve blood pressure goals due to their ability to preserve kidney function. Hydrochlorothiazide is also considered a first line agent to treat hypertension; however, the dose should be limited to less than 25 mg daily to avoid worsening insulin resistance (C).

7. **B.** The question's focus is on assessment and screening for eating disorders, of which intentional insulin omission is one. Her elevated A1C in light of her concern that her boyfriend is interested in a thinner woman are clues that she may be intentionally omitting her insulin for weight control purposes. Effective assessments reveal lifestyle issues and facts, are patient centered, and facilitate honest self-disclosure. They identify needs of the individual and factors that interfere with an individual's activities of daily living. Effective assessments find the high-priority problems to be solved.

    Fear should not be used to try to motivate (A). Scare tactics are actually counterproductive, leading an individual to withdraw from the interaction, stop listening, and abandon the relationship.

    Furthermore, this is an adult, and whether or not her parents are aware of her poor blood glucose control really isn't an issue (C).

    Asking the time of day that she checks her blood glucose would not offer useful information given the degree of elevation of her A1C, indicating general poor blood glucose control. The underlying issue is inadequate insulin dosing (D).

8. **B.** A blood glucose level between 100 and 125 mg/dL indicates impaired fasting glucose. A normal fasting blood glucose is <100 mg/dL and diabetes is indicated by a fasting blood sugar of ≥126 mg/dL, making A and C incorrect choices. Since there is no mention that the individual is pregnant, D is also not the correct choice.

121

Review Guide for the CDE® Exam

9. **B.**   Peripheral arterial disease is correct. Swelling and redness when the feet hang down are signs of poor circulation and peripheral vascular disease. Diabetic neuropathy (A) may accompany peripheral vascular disease; however, these visually observable changes are not usually present. Varicose veins (C) and Charcot joint (D) are also not usual causes of foot swelling and redness.

10. **A.**   This question is addressing setting learning objectives, as opposed to behavioral objectives. While all of these answers might seem like appropriate actions that the patient could take, only one is actually a learning objective.

A *learning objective* (also known as an educational objective) is what the participant is expected to meet at the completion of a teaching session. Learning objectives provide a basis for making the best possible inferences about whether learning occurred.

A *behavioral objective* is a planned change in behavior that is expected to result in improved health or quality of life. It's a behavior under the participant's direct control that is selected by and/or written by the participant. Behavior objectives are SMART—Specific, Measurable, Achievable, Realistic, and Time-bound.

Both learning and behavioral objectives are written as measurable, observable statements so the participant and educator can clearly determine if objectives have been met. Answers B, C, and D are incorrect as they are behavioral objectives—they meet the SMART criteria.

11. **C.**   Strong evidence shows that replacing saturated fats and trans fats (the most atherogenic types of fats) in the diet with unsaturated fats (mono- and polyunsaturated fats) lowers both total cholesterol and LDL cholesterol.

Studies have not demonstrated a reduction in total and LDL cholesterol with a weight loss of 3–5%. More recent studies in individuals with diabetes have shown positive effects on TG and HDL, but not with LDL and total cholesterol with even a 5–10% weight loss (A).

Studies have not demonstrated a reduction in LDL and total cholesterol with resistance exercise twice/week (B).

Although red wine has been shown to have cardiovascular benefits, there has not been conclusive evidence to show a reduction in LDL and total cholesterol. In addition, a moderate alcohol intake is defined as 1 drink/day for women, not 2 (D).

12. **D.**   This question is addressing her anxiety and consideration of an appropriate referral.

Answer D is correct. MN has been experiencing generalized anxiety and may benefit from consultation with a mental health professional to assist in managing the anxiety and resulting overeating.

Section 4: Answer Key

As no cardiac concerns are noted, consultation with a cardiologist is not necessary at this time. MN's significantly elevated lipids are a relatively new concern. Lifestyle modification as a first step may help improve the lipid profile (A).

There is no indication of renal concerns requiring referral to a nephrologist (B).

There is no indication of social/financial concerns requiring referral to a social worker (C).

13. **B.** Assessment is the first step in the process of providing diabetes education. By understanding what the interests, needs, and problems of the person with diabetes are, the educator is more likely to provide appropriate and useful information that will assist the individual to meet desired outcomes. The other choices, understanding of pathophysiology (A), chronic complications (C), and carbohydrate counting (D), may well become part of the education plan, but this follows assessment.

14. **D.** HMG-CoA reductase inhibitors is correct. Statin drugs are category X and should not be used in pregnant women. Human insulin (A), metformin (B), and methyldopa (C) have adequate safety data to support use during pregnancy.

15. **A.** When verifying the accuracy of a meter, the blood glucose meter results should be compared against a laboratory value, not another meter. Only fasting values can be compared since postmeal values will differ between the capillary blood (as measured on the meter) and the venous blood (as measured in the lab).

When comparing a meter result with a lab result, the 2 tests must be done at the same time. Measuring blood glucose at home either before or after the venipuncture allows too much time between the readings for a valid comparison (B).

The meter result would be ~15% LOWER than the laboratory result if the meter reports whole blood glucose values (C).

Comparing meter readings with lab values involves a fingertip or alternate site puncture AND a venipuncture. Applying a drop of blood from the venipuncture needle is not acceptable, as the meter strips will give false readings if venous blood is used (D).

16. **C.** Ketone testing is appropriate during illness, when blood glucose levels are consistently elevated, and during weight loss and pregnancy. It does not need to be done daily (A), prior to a decrease in insulin dose (B), or prior to exercise unless glucoses are elevated, making this choice incorrect (D).

17. **C.** Other developmental characteristics of this group are greater experimentation and risk taking; physical and social activity increases; opposite sex relationships emerge and are important; and formal operational thinking begins, along with abstract reasoning.

Answer A is a characteristic of late adolescence (age 16–21 years). Answer B is incorrect. This is a characteristic of early adolescence (age 12 years). Answer D is incorrect. This is a characteristic of late adolescence (age 16–21 years).

123

Review Guide for the CDE® Exam

18. **C.** Role-playing is an active form of teaching and learning that allows the learner to practice, express, explore, discuss, and share. Role-playing facilitates exploration of "what if" situations. This format can be useful in an individual or group setting.

    Games allow for interactive learning, but are not the best venue for practicing, expressing, and exploring strategies for dealing with peer pressure (A).

    The goal of discussion is to seek and acquire information rather than practicing dealing with "what if" situations (B).

    Lecturing is a passive form of learning and just allows for the presentation of information. It would not allow for LJ to explore and practice dealing with peer pressure situations (D).

19. **A.** Answer A is correct and answers B, C, and D are incorrect. The duration of the honeymoon period varies, but typically lasts between 3 and 12 months.

20. **B.** Effective assessments should reveal potential barriers to self-management. Financial concerns and a lack of adequate insurance represent a major obstacle to care and therefore would be the appropriate place to begin. For patients with health insurance prescription coverage, the copayment does not change among pharmacy chains (A) or without notice (C). Copayments for 3-month supplies of medications are typically less than 3 times a one-month supply (D).

21. **B.** The focus of this question is on assessing lifestyle effects on the diabetes treatment plan. The key problem is time pressure and diabetes treatment plan complexity.

    This patient has a hectic schedule with family commitments, complicated further by a complex medication plan with 4 diabetes medications. The many demands on her time likely make adhering to her diabetes treatment plan difficult. The educator will want to explore contributors to the patient's fluctuating glucose control, particularly how many medication doses are missed. She could certainly benefit from simplification of her diabetes treatment plan.

    While she may gain some improvement in blood glucose from an increase in her bedtime glargine, the real question is whether she's actually taking all of her prescribed medication doses currently. Furthermore, it's unlikely that she'll have time to monitor blood glucose more frequently, if that's even necessary (A).

    Insulin pump therapy would be more labor intensive for this patient than her current plan (C).

    Keeping a 3-month food diary would be an unreasonable request for this patient (nor is it even necessary) given the many demands she already has on her time (D).

22. **D.** The National Standards for Diabetes Self-Management Education and Support specify in Standard 5 that at least one of the program's instructors must be a registered nurse, dietitian, or pharmacist.

124

Section 4: Answer Key

23. **A.** Contact the local pharmacy that fills her prescriptions is correct. The local pharmacy will be able to provide objective data and estimates of long-term adherence. Podiatrists (B) may collect some medication history, but it is unlikely to be complete. Because the patient lives in an assisted living environment, her daughter is unlikely to be able to provide useful information regarding daily care, especially while she is at work (C). Drug pictures in the Physicians' Desk Reference (D) may be useful for some drugs; however, generic products often are not listed.

24. **B.** The educational process always begins with assessment, ie, in this case understanding why the patient does not want to start insulin. The other choices assume what the problem—lack of knowledge (A), fear of pain (C), and experiences of family members (D)—may be without involving the patient in the process and therefore are not correct choices.

25. **C.** The blood glucose values are not accurate is correct. Clues to fabricated home blood glucose values include daily testing at exactly the same time without missed days, absence of blood smears on the pages with neatly written numbers in the same ink, frequently repeated values, and values all within the desired range. The A1C for this patient would be expected to fall less than 7% based on the home readings (A and B). Food does not affect the A1C, making it very reproducible in the same patient (D).

26. **B.** These are all symptoms of depression. Weight loss with an eating disorder would be intentional (A). With an anxiety disorder (C), the major symptoms include sweating, tremulousness, weakness, lack of concentration, irritability, and restlessness, making this choice incorrect. Anger would be characterized by outbursts, making anger management (D) an incorrect choice.

27. **B.** Honest self-disclosure occurs only when people trust each other. The educator's task is to develop an atmosphere of trust and to do so quickly.

    This comment could destroy JT's trust in the educator and any rapport that's been built. The educator's goal is to maintain an attitude of nonjudgmental acceptance, which means listening, repeating, and asking more questions while avoiding criticism, sarcasm, horror, stereotyping, or disgust. The educator strives to learn of people's problems, progress, and successes, not to pass judgment on them (A).

    Scare tactics are actually counterproductive, leading an individual to withdraw from the interaction, stop listening, and abandon the relationship (C).

    Monitoring blood glucose twice a month is not adequate to assess blood glucose control, particularly since her blood glucose is around 200 mg/dL when she DOES check it (D).

28. **A.** Precontemplation is correct. This patient has not begun to consider the need to check her blood glucose more often. This essential step precedes contemplation of the change value (B) and preparation (C) of the necessary elements to begin the change. The action stage (D) in this patient would be identified by more frequent blood glucose testing.

125

Review Guide for the CDE® Exam

29. **B.** B is the correct answer because the educational process always begins with assessment. In this case understanding why the patient is not monitoring blood glucose is an initial step. The other choices make assumptions regarding the cause of the problem (A—healthy eating, C—taking medication, and D—being active) without involving the patient in the process and therefore are not the best choices.

30. **D.** The focus of this question is on assessment, specifically assessment of the patient's psychomotor skills.

Demonstration of an injection by the educator, then return demonstration by the patient, allows for active learning. It allows the learner to observe, perform, and receive evaluation of their technique. The educator is able to assess whether the patient is able to correctly perform self-injection or whether injections will need to be performed by a caretaker (D).

Asking the patient to describe injection steps would provide some assessment of cognitive capabilities, but not patient's motor skills and capability of correctly injecting (A). Asking the patient to write out the procedure does not provide assessment of psychomotor skills related to injection technique (B).

Providing a pamphlet on injection technique does not provide any assessment of patient's actual ability to correctly inject (C).

31. **D.** Most adults who are illiterate have learned to hide their literacy deficit and manage to compensate for this deficit and function in society. People do not tend to reveal that they are illiterate (A). The number of years of schooling completed is not an indicator of literacy level (B). The types of newspapers and magazines that a person reads is not an indicator of his or her literacy level (C).

32. **C.** By definition, role-playing is a form of active learning that allows the learner to practice, express, explore, discuss, and share. Answers A, B, and D are incorrect.

33. **D.** According to adult learning theory, adults learn best when they feel the need to know, when it is personally relevant, and when it is active. A, B, and C are incorrect because they do not involve the patient in the process.

34. **B.** The focus of this question is on assessing needs and making referrals as appropriate. College students by nature have variable schedules and typically variable food intake from day to day. The fact that this student takes the same insulin dose with each meal, despite carbohydrate intake, does not maximize her diabetes control.

This patient could benefit from a consult with a registered dietitian for education on carbohydrate counting and using insulin-to-carbohydrate ratios.

While the patient could gain some valuable information on meal planning from the Internet, the information is not individualized for her needs, nor does she have the opportunity to ask questions and receive feedback as with a personal consult (A).

SECTION 4: ANSWER KEY

126

Section 4: Answer Key

Although family support is important, the key issue is carbohydrate counting, which the patient must understand and be able to implement on her own (C).

Written materials do not replace individualized nutrition education by a registered dietitian (D).

35. **B.** An insulin sensitivity factor of 31 is correct. The insulin sensitivity factor or correction bolus determines the amount of glucose lowering expected from 1 unit of insulin. In this patient, on multiple daily injections with glargine and rapid-acting insulin, the calculation is as follows: 1,700 divided by the total daily dose of insulin (55 units in this case). Historically, this calculation used 1,500 in the numerator; however, 1,700 provides a more accurate estimate. Therefore, each of the other responses is incorrect (A, C, and D).

36. **B.** A registered dietitian is the most appropriate referral for PW. He is motivated to control his blood glucose, but has expressed concern about weight gain. A registered dietitian can teach him how to avoid weight gain on his new insulin regimen. None of the other healthcare professionals suggested would be appropriate choices in this situation (A, C, D).

37. **B.** Increasing the frequency of blood glucose monitoring is important for sick-day management because the signs and symptoms of a developing acute illness can be preceded by elevated blood glucose levels and ketone levels.

Insulin doses should continue as able and adjusted to correct hyperglycemia (A). Individuals should drink beverages with 15 g carbohydrate-containing liquids (C).

Healthcare professionals should be contacted when the individual has episodes of vomiting, diarrhea, or elevated blood glucose levels that are not responsive to insulin and fluids or has moderate or large urine ketones or blood ketones >0.6 mmol/L (D).

38. **C.** The stem has all the characteristics of a behavioral objective. It is specific, measurable, achievable, realistic, and time bound, and it represents a planned change in behavior. A learning objective relates to the completion of a teaching session, although learning objectives are also measurable (B). A goal is the big-picture, directional guide. It is the focal point for and the end results of meeting the learning and behavioral objectives (D). An assessment is conducted by the educator to gather sufficient information about the patient to help identify goals and an individual education plan (A).

39. **B.** SMART is a simple acronym to guide educators in assessing the completeness of their behavioral objectives. A behavioral objective is a planned change in behavior that is expected to result in improved health or quality of life.

Answers A, C, and D are incorrect because SMART is not applicable to a learning objective, action plan, or evaluation.

Review Guide for the CDE® Exam

40. **C.** Methods of instruction that focus on non-print media are more effective for individuals with low literacy skills. The other responses (A, B, and D) are incorrect because they do not represent effective teaching strategies.

41. **B.** The primary nutrition goal for individuals with type 1 diabetes is to establish an insulin plan that fits into their preferred eating routine and lifestyle. The total and type of carbohydrate in meals and snacks directly affect blood glucose levels, so this is the primary area of focus. Those individuals on a fixed insulin plan should strive for consistency in carbohydrate intake, while those on a flexible insulin plan or insulin pump should adjust their insulin and food based on their insulin-to-carbohydrate ratio. As a result, B is the correct answer and answers A, C, and D are incorrect.

42. **D.** Computers is correct. Appropriately designed computer programs are well suited for on-demand, self-directed learning. Discussions (A) with patients are useful, but may not be as convenient as computer resources. Print materials (B) are useful to convey information, but tend to be very linear in their presentation. Computer programs are often designed to repeat sections where patients do not perform up to certain expectations. Role-playing (C) is also useful to reinforce problem-solving strategies, but may not be convenient for patients with busy schedules.

43. **B.** The focus of this question is appropriate referral.

    The Gestational Diabetes Mellitus (GDM) Evidence Based Nutrition Practice Guidelines state that it is imperative for women diagnosed with GDM to be referred to a registered dietitian within 48 hours of diagnosis and have medical nutrition therapy (MNT) implemented within 1 week of diagnosis (B, C, D).

    The need for initiation of MNT following diagnosis of GDM is not weight driven (A). The Nutrition Practice Guidelines state that all women with GDM should consult with a registered dietitian within 1 week of diagnosis, and include a minimum of 3 nutrition visits. There is strong research evidence indicating that MNT results in improved maternal and neonatal outcomes, particularly when GDM is diagnosed and treated early.

44. **C.** SP's prepregnancy BMI was in the "overweight" category (BMI >26.0–29.0).

    According to the Institute of Medicine (IOM), corresponding recommended weight gain in pregnancy for a woman with a prepregnancy BMI in the "overweight" category is 15–25 lbs (C). The other responses are the IOM's recommended weight gain for a woman with a prepregnancy "underweight" BMI of <19.8 (A), a woman with a prepregnancy "normal weight" BMI of 19.8–26.0 (B), and a woman with a prepregnancy "obese" BMI of >29.0 (D).

45. **C.** Needle anxiety occurs in almost everyone to varying degrees. If severe or persistent and left unresolved, diabetes control may suffer because of missed injections, inadequate testing, and avoidance of healthcare follow-up visits. A skilled diabetes educator will

Section 4: Answer Key

learn to match and individualize the presentation of the BG monitoring so that the fears of the person with diabetes may be alleviated.

46. **D.** Role-playing is an active form of learning that facilitates the sharing of information and therefore works well in a group setting. Although the use of computer simulation programs (B) is also an active form of learning, they target individuals rather than a group. Lectures (A) and the distribution of learning materials (C) can provide information, but they both are passive learning experiences and do not draw on the real-life experiences of the group participants.

47. **D.** According to the American Diabetes Association's (ADA's) Clinical Practice Recommendations: Diagnosis and Classification of Diabetes Mellitus, the criteria for diagnosis of diabetes are as follows:

   • Fasting plasma glucose ≥126 mg/dL OR
   • Symptoms of hyperglycemia and a casual plasma glucose ≥200 mg/dL OR
   • 2-hour plasma glucose ≥200 mg/dL during a 75-gram oral glucose tolerance test.

   Answer D is correct as these parameters meet the criteria for diagnosis of diabetes.

   Polyuria is a symptom of hyperglycemia, but cannot be used as a diagnostic criterion for diabetes (A). An A1C of 5.1–6.4% would be diagnostic of prediabetes (B).

   A fasting plasma glucose 100–125 mg/dL is indicative of impaired fasting glucose (C).

48. **C.** Diabetes can also be diagnosed by acute symptoms plus casual plasma glucose >200 mg/dL or by OGTT testing (2 hr >200 mg/dL). The HLA genotype is strongly associated with the occurrence of type 1 diabetes but again is not diagnostic (B). Although some individuals are diagnosed with type 1 diabetes when they develop DKA, it is not a criterion for diagnosis (D).

49. **A.** The focus of this question is normal fuel homeostasis, which occurs in 5 phases.

   Phase II of fuel homeostasis is the postabsorptive state. During this phase, blood glucose originates from glycogen breakdown and hepatic gluconeogenesis. Plasma insulin levels decrease and glucagon levels begin to rise. Energy storage ends and energy production begins. Carbohydrate and lipid stores are mobilized. Hepatic glycogen breakdown provides maintenance of plasma glucose and ensures an adequate supply of glucose for the brain and other tissues. Adipocyte triglyceride begins to break down and free fatty acids are released into circulation and used by the liver and skeletal muscle as a primary energy source and as a substrate for gluconeogenesis. The brain continues to use glucose, provided mainly by gluconeogenesis, because of its inability to use free fatty acids as fuel.

   Insulin inhibits breakdown of glycogen and triglyceride reservoirs during Phase I (B).

   Counter-regulatory hormone secretion is stimulated during Phase IV (C). Excess glucose is stored in hepatic, muscle, adipose, and other tissue reservoirs during Phase I (D).

Review Guide for the CDE® Exam

50. **A.** LT displays several common symptoms of depression including lack of interest (has stopped glucose monitoring), sleep disturbances, and difficulty concentrating. Mental health issues such as depression may interfere with diabetes self-management and diabetes control and therefore should be addressed first.

51. **C.** This question focuses on teaching strategies and the learning experience. Demonstration, an active form of learning, is the most effective teaching strategy to teach this psychomotor skill. It allows for the educator to demonstrate correct monitoring technique and for the patient to provide return demonstration. This teaching strategy allows the learner to observe, perform, and be evaluated.

Lecture is a passive form of learning and does not allow the educator to evaluate the learner's ability to actually perform self-monitoring of blood glucose (A).

An online presentation does not allow for discussion between the educator and the patient or demonstration of skills in order for the educator to observe and evaluate the patient's ability to use the meter (B).

The patient has already reviewed the instruction manual (print materials). Other print materials cannot replace in-person education with demonstration and return demonstration for the educator to assess the patient's self-monitoring of blood glucose skills (D).

52. **B.** Preparation is correct. This patient has considered the value of testing his blood glucose (A) and made necessary preparations to take action; however, he has yet to complete the task (C). Repetition of the testing process would be classified as maintenance (D).

53. **A.** Successful completion of a task helps to increase self-efficacy. The educator supports the behavior change by providing positive feedback on the performance of the behavior. Choices B, C, and D are incorrect because they do not focus on the behavior of interest.

54. **C.** Early type 1 diabetes is first identified by the appearance of active autoimmunity directed against pancreatic beta cells and their products. Glutamic acid decarboxylase (GAD) appears to be the best immunologic predictor for the future development of type 1 diabetes (C). These islet cell antibodies may play a permissive or pathologic role in the causation of type 1 diabetes, but are not the best predictor (A, B, and D).

55. **C.** Type 2 diabetes is correct. Although many patients are diagnosed with type 2 diabetes based on 2 fasting plasma glucose values above 126 mg/dL, patients with hyperglycemic symptoms may also be diagnosed with a random plasma glucose value above 200 mg/dL. Impaired fasting glucose (A) is defined as values between 100 and 125 mg/dL, whereas impaired glucose tolerance is defined as a 2-hour postprandial plasma glucose above 140 mg/dL but less than 200 mg/dL (D). The age of the patient and absence of ketones with this degree of elevated plasma glucose are not consistent with type 1 diabetes (B).

SECTION 4: ANSWER KEY

Section 4: Answer Key

56. **B.**   CMS currently reimburses for 10 program hours of initial diabetes education and 2 hours in each subsequent year. (Source: Diabetes Self-management Education and Support in Type 2 Diabetes: A Joint Position Statement of the American Diabetes Association, the American Association of Diabetes Educators, and the Academy of Nutrition and Dietetics)

57. **C.**   A normal oral glucose tolerance test (A) would be characterized by a 1-hour peak less than 180 mg/dL and a return to less than 140 mg/dL after 3 hours. This test demonstrated consistently elevated blood glucose levels throughout the evaluation period (B). This patient does not have type 1 diabetes, as evidenced by her ability to maintain a normal fasting blood glucose level (D).

58. **B.**   Adjustment disorder with depressed mood is defined by the American Psychiatric Association (APA) as the development of depressive symptoms (eg, sleeping after school, withdrawing from friends) within a 3-month period of time following a stressor (eg, not being selected for the cheerleading squad). With this disorder, depressive symptoms cause impairment in social, occupational, or other areas of functioning OR are in excess of what would be expected from exposure to the stressor. Symptoms are expected to remit within 6 months of the time of onset.

    Unintentional changes in weight or appetite are characteristic of major depressive disorder or dysthymic disorder (A). Early morning awakening for at least 1 week is characteristic of major depressive disorder (C). Presence of manic symptoms is not characteristic of adjustment disorder with depressed mood (D).

59. **A.**   This question is focusing on nutrition assessment, step 1 of the Nutrition Care Process. As for assessment of food and nutrition history, relevant data to be gathered include 24-hour recall or typical day's food intake with specific details on eating times, alcohol intake, and the use of vitamins, minerals, and herbal supplements.

    The sick-day plan, insurance coverage, and family support are not components of the nutrition assessment (B, C, and D).

60. **C.**   By definition, instrumental support is providing concrete assistance, such as GG's neighbor helping him with his medications and blood glucose monitoring. Instrumental support is the type of support most individuals are referring to when they talk about "help."

    Emotional support involves caring, empathy, love, and trust. While GG's neighbor could possibly provide some emotional support as well, instrumental support is clearly what's described in the scenario (A). Informational support is provision of information to another during a time of stress (B). Affirmational support is statements that affirm the appropriateness of acts or statement of another (D).

131

Review Guide for the CDE® Exam

61. **A.** A number of meal planning approaches are available to teach basic diabetes nutrition guidelines, as well as more in-depth nutrition interventions. Of the 4 meal planning resources listed here, given GG's cognitive limitations, the plate method would be the most appropriate because it uses a simple dinner plate graphic to teach general portion control, consistency, and basic food categories.

    Carbohydrate counting (B) and the exchange lists (C) would be too complicated given GG's cognitive limitations. The DASH eating plan (D) is not as simple as the plate method and would not be the best choice for that reason.

62. **C.** "What is it that concerns you most about starting insulin?" is correct. The educator should seek first to understand patient concerns from the patient himself rather than imposing predetermined values. In answers A and B, the educator presumes to know why the patient is concerned before finding out the real, underlying reason. Both assumptions present close-ended questions to the patient. Answer D suggests that the patient may have used illicit drugs in the past, which the patient may or may not answer truthfully.

63. **B.** This question focuses on assessment of diabetes self-care considering age-related traits of youth and delegation of diabetes care responsibilities. Youth ages 12–15 years are increasingly more independent. The caregiver's responsibility is to continue delegation of diabetes self-management tasks and to provide physical and mental health support as needed.

    Developmentally, a 14-year-old is able to administer his or her own insulin (A). A 14-year-old is capable of planning foods to be consumed at each meal/snack. It's particularly important that the individual is able to plan foods to be consumed since he or she is spending more time away from home and becoming more responsible for his or her actions (C). At age 5–8 years, children may actually be able to perform self-monitoring of blood glucose independently (D).

64. **C.** The Centers for Disease Control and Prevention recommends that individuals with diabetes see a dentist every 6 months and more often if periodontal disease is present.

65. **B.** Adjustment disorder with depressed mood is correct. This patient reports an identifiable cause of her depression. Major depressive disorder (A) and dysthymic disorder (C) are not associated with an identifiable cause of the psychological response. This patient's adjustment disorder is characterized by tearfulness, which is consistent with depression, rather than nervousness, worry, or jitteriness expected with anxiety (D).

66. **B.** Bingeing (excessive food intake with an accompanying sense of loss of control) is the most commonly reported disordered eating behavior in individuals with type 2 diabetes. Purging, anorexia nervosa, and insulin omission to facilitate weight loss are more commonly reported among people with type 1 diabetes (A, C, D).

SECTION 4: ANSWER KEY

Section 4: Answer Key

67. **B.** Hypoglycemia is correct. The combination of exercise, delayed eating, and a sulfonyl-urea increases the likelihood of hypoglycemia. Resolution of these symptoms with food further eliminates hyperglycemia (A), overexertion (C), and ketoacidosis (D) as possible causes.

68. **C.** Self-monitored blood glucose lets patients see how food affects their glycemic control is correct. Patients who reach their glycemic goals on oral drug therapy only need to test their blood glucose a few times each week (A). Patients who are poorly controlled, changing therapy, or on insulin should test their blood glucose levels at least 1 or 2 times daily (B). Urine testing is not appropriate to monitor or adjust drug therapy (D).

69. **A.** Operator technique is correct. Inaccurate results from self-monitoring of blood glucose can come from a variety of sources; however, the most common is operator technique. Many newer blood glucose meters are self-calibrating (B) and do not start the test until an adequate sample is applied (D). Using expired or defective test strips may also cause inaccurate results; however, newer testing methodologies make this error less significant (C).

70. **B.** Persons taking a TZD should be told that the maximum glucose-lowering effect of these medications may not be apparent until after 8 to 12 weeks of use. Since the patient only has been on a TZD for 1 month, it is a logical first step to wait to see if the medications have an effect on glucose levels before looking to make changes in diet and exercise (A and D) or referring the patient back to the doctor for the addition of another oral agent (C).

71. **A.** The basal insulin dose controls blood glucose levels in between meals when the individual is not eating. Therefore, fasting blood glucose data is the best indicator of the appropriateness of the basal insulin dose. During the day, patients may choose to skip a meal to treat the appropriateness of a basal insulin dose. Postprandial glucose levels best reflect the effect of the bolus insulin regimen, making B, C, and D incorrect.

72. **D.** Use a blood glucose meter with alternate site testing capabilities is correct. Although a glucose sensor may be useful to augment capillary testing, the sensors must be calibrated each day with several finger-sticks (A). Because stress can affect blood glucose, this patient may need to test more often before a concert to appropriately adjust his insulin dose (B). Urine testing is not appropriate to replace blood glucose testing in patients with diabetes (C).

73. **C.** According to the ADA Standards of Medical Care, if systolic blood pressure is ≥140 mm Hg or diastolic ≥90 mm Hg, blood pressure should be confirmed on a separate day. Repeat systolic blood pressure ≥140 mm Hg or diastolic ≥90 mm Hg confirms a diagnosis of hypertension. Answer A is incorrect for the reasons noted above. Blood pressure should be confirmed promptly to determine a course of intervention, if necessary (B). The ADA Standards of Medical Care state that individuals with a confirmed blood pressure of >140/90 mm Hg, in addition to lifestyle therapy, should have prompt initiation of pharmacologic agents (D).

133

Review Guide for the CDE® Exam

74. **C.** Assessment is the first step in the process of providing diabetes education. By understanding what the interests, needs, and problems of the person with diabetes are, the educator is more likely to provide appropriate and useful information that will assist the individual to meet desired outcomes. Healthcare system issues are not germane to this visit (A). Both B and D are important issues to cover but do not need to occur in the first visit.

75. **C.** The meal plan definitely must meet the energy requirements for growth and activity.

    The term "food plan" or "meal plan" should be used rather than "diet" to avoid negative connotations (A).

    Nutrition education to promote healthy eating for children and adolescents should involve the entire family and caretakers, and be geared toward the appropriate developmental stage of the child. A 12-year-old is capable of providing input on foods for meals/snacks (B).

    One key area of focus in meal plans for children and adolescents is the inclusion of nutrient-dense foods (D).

76. **D.** This question tests assessment skills. Key information noted includes improved blood glucose, significant weight loss, continuation of 3 meals each day, and no change in physical activity. Beverage choices could significantly impact blood glucose and weight via reduced carbohydrate and calorie intake.

    Omission of glipizide would lead to deterioration in blood glucose control, rather than improved blood glucose control as noted (A).

    While over-the-counter supplement and medication use is an area to assess, taking a multivitamin would not affect weight or blood glucose (B).

    Reducing screen time could result in increased activity, but not likely enough to result in a 10-lb weight loss and significantly improved blood glucose control (C).

77. **B.** A pedometer records steps/day, a lifestyle activity. Other forms of monitors are unrelated to lifestyle activity (A, C, and D). Blood glucose meters monitor blood glucose levels, a blood pressure cuff and meter monitors blood pressure, and a Holter monitor monitors cardiac rhythms.

78. **D.** The Dietary Guidelines for Americans recommend at least 60 minutes of moderate-intensity physical activity daily for children and adolescents (D).

    When addressing lifestyle intervention in children and adolescents, the focus must be one of substitution and reduction rather than elimination. Instead of recommending avoidance of fast food, the suggestion might be to learn to make healthier choices at fast-food restaurants (A).

    Again, for success, the focus must be on reduction rather than elimination. A more realistic suggestion would be to reduce consumption of fatty, calorie-dense foods (B).

SECTION 4: ANSWER KEY

134

Section 4: Answer Key

While physical activity would certainly lower insulin resistance and help maintain weight loss, overweight and obese youths often lack the stamina and athletic ability to compete in sports. Physical activities can be a source of self-degradation and ridicule by peers, contributing to poor self-esteem. Rather than focusing on competitive sports, the child should be encouraged to improve fitness through individual activities like biking or skating (C).

79. **C.** By definition, 1 carbohydrate choice equals 15 grams carbohydrate. One serving of this food contains 16 grams carbohydrate, so 2 servings contain 32 grams carbohydrate, which is 2 carbohydrate choices (or servings).

80. **B.** In the Diabetes Prevention Program study, patients at risk for diabetes were randomized to lifestyle modification (B), metformin (D), or placebo. A thiazolidinedione arm was initially included using the drug troglitazone, but was discontinued due to liver toxicity (A). Patients in the lifestyle modification group experienced a 58% reduction in diabetes progression, compared with a 31% reduction in the metformin group.

81. **A.** Other food sources of monounsaturated fats include avocados, almonds, pecans, and peanuts. When substituted for saturated fats, monounsaturated fats can decrease LDL cholesterol and triglyceride levels without decreasing HDL cholesterol.

82. **D.** Assessment of the target population should include ethnic background, formal education level, reading ability, and barriers to participation in education. The assessment should not be limited to individuals who frequently attend medical appointments (B), but encompass all individuals with diabetes. Knowledge about diabetes and its complications is not an assessment criterion (A). Social or family support is not a criterion for assessing the target population (C).

83. **A.** Individuals with cardiac disease must focus particular attention on blood pressure and heart rate response during resistance training. The heart rate and blood pressure need to remain within the limits established by an exercise stress test and, therefore, need to be monitored throughout the training session. Starting with lighter resistance and choosing exercises that use a smaller amount of muscle mass help decrease the myocardial oxygen demand on the heart.

In the absence of contraindications, all patients with diabetes should be encouraged to engage in resistance training at least twice each week. Recommended duration of resistance training is 1 to 3 sets of 8–20 repetitions. Aerobic exercise is important, but patients with osteopenia benefit most from resistance training. Aerobic exercise has not been shown to result in the same bone-strengthening benefits as resistance exercises (B).

When performing resistance training, individuals with cardiovascular disease should be advised to breathe continually and avoid breath holding. They should exhale during the exertion or lifting phase and inhale while returning to starting position (C).

The recommendation is to lift weights with slow, controlled movements. One should stop exercising if warning signs or symptoms of cardiac distress occur, such as dizziness, unusual shortness of breath, or chest pain (D).

Review Guide for the CDE® Exam

84. **D.** One of the first steps in the development of a new education program is to assess the target population and determine their educational needs. Choices A, B, and C are incorrect because they need to occur later in the process once the program is developed and ready to be implemented.

85. **B.** The physical activity guideline for obese individuals is 45–60 minutes of moderate-intensity physical activity 5–7 days per week.

Answer A is incorrect. A combination of physical activity, meal planning, and behavior change has proven to be most effective for obese individuals. Physical activity in combination with meal planning has been shown to be more effective for long-term weight loss than either alone. Physical activity offers enhanced calorie expenditure and improved fitness in terms of influencing blood lipids, blood glucose control, blood pressure, mood, and attitude. Regular physical activity also helps maintain muscle mass while promoting fat loss during weight loss (A).

Swimming is actually LESS likely to induce weight loss (C).

The recommendation is to advise moderate-intensity activities with emphasis on increasing duration and frequency. Intensity can be progressively increased to improve aerobic capacity, but is not necessary if lower intensity is preferred (D).

86. **B.** Six months following the initial diagnosis of type 2 diabetes is not one of the four critical times to assess, adjust, provide, and refer a patient for DSMES. The four critical times are (1) at diagnosis, (2) annually, (3) when new complicating factors influence self-management, and (4) when transitions of care occur. Transitions of care include changes in the patient's living situation, medical care team, insurance coverage resulting in treatment change, age-related changes affecting cognition, self-care, etc.

87. **D.** Literacy is a factor that influences learning. Hearing (A), visual acuity (B), and mobility (C) are physical factors.

88. **C.** Worsening of hyperglycemia and ketosis can occur in the presence of absolute insulin deficiency. As a rule of thumb, ketone levels should be checked with blood glucose levels above 250 mg/dL. If ketones are present, then the elevated blood glucose level is a result of insulin deficiency and corrective action should be taken immediately. In the absence of ketones, this higher value should not pose a medical threat; however, some people experience headaches, blurry vision, or lack of energy with higher blood glucose results, which are reasons in themselves to avoid physical activity until blood glucose level improves.

The concern in this scenario is existing hyperglycemia. Consuming a snack would only drive blood glucose higher (A).

Physical activity performed at intense aerobic levels can result in blood glucose levels climbing higher in type 1 diabetes, particularly in the presence of insulin deficiency (B) and (D).

136

Section 4: Answer Key

89. **B.** Although Medicare regulations dictate that most patients receive their education in a group setting in order to qualify for reimbursement, the following are exceptions: No group session is available within 2 months of the date education is ordered; the individual has severe vision, language, or hearing limitations or other conditions identified by the treating healthcare provider (A, C, and D).

90. **B.** Low-fat or skim milk is correct. Acarbose inhibits the enzyme alpha-glucosidase, which is responsible for breaking down complex carbohydrates in the proximal portion of the small intestines. Lactose is not affected by acarbose, so milk is absorbed at its normal rate. Fructose and sucrose found in orange juice (A), hard candy (C), and regular soda (D) would all experience delayed metabolism in the presence of acarbose.

91. **C.** All levels of documentation are protected under the Health Insurance Portability and Accountability Act. Personal health information must always be stored, analyzed, and reported in a manner that protects the identification of individuals.

92. **B.** Inhibition of hepatic glucose release is correct. Each of the other answers describes the main mechanism of action of other drug classes. Thiazolidinediones improve insulin sensitivity in skeletal muscle (A). Alpha-glucosidase inhibitors delay absorption of carbohydrates from the GI tract (C). Sulfonylureas and meglitinides enhance insulin secretion from the islet cells of the pancreas (D).

93. **A.** Meglitinides is correct. Although less likely than longer-acting insulin secretagogues, meglitinides are more likely to cause hypoglycemia than other oral agents. Thiazolidinediones (B), biguanides (C), and DPP-IV inhibitors (D) are not likely to cause hypoglycemia and would be better choices for this active patient.

94. **A.** A QI process is a systemic review of process and outcome data to measure the effectiveness of the education and support and looks for ways to improve any identified gaps in service or service quality. The process includes staff from a variety of levels and departments that are relevant to the specific QI project (B). A QI project can select a number of groups as the customer, including patients with diabetes, third-party payors, regulatory agencies, etc. (C). Implementing a QI process in a DSME program is recommended in Standard 10 of the National Standards (D).

95. **A.** Use of contraception is correct. Resolution of hyperglycemia with metformin in patients with polycystic ovarian syndrome often restores menstruation and ability to become pregnant. Thiazolidinediones and biguanides are not associated with hypoglycemia (B). This patient is not at risk for ketoacidosis because she has type 2 diabetes (C). Dilsulfiram-like reactions are associated with first generation sulfonylureas, but not with this patient's regimen (D).

Review Guide for the CDE® Exam

96. **D.** With insulin pump therapy the dawn phenomenon effects are easier to manage because a variable basal rate can be set to accommodate fluctuations in insulin requirements overnight. Basal rates can be lowered during periods of low physiological requirements, which can minimize nocturnal or daytime hypoglycemia. Carbohydrate counting (A), increased basal dose (B), and more frequent blood glucose monitoring (C) could all help to improve glucose control and may offer improvement but not to the same degree as insulin pump therapy.

97. **A.** A blood glucose level greater than 600 mg/dL, without significant ketones, characterizes hyperosmolar hyperglycemic state (HHS). Extreme dehydration, more than profound insulin deficiency, is the primary precipitating factor. HHS develops slowly and does not cause the gastrointestinal pain and Kussmaul respirations associated with DKA (B).

98. **B.** This question addresses lifestyle interventions to help prevent type 2 diabetes in overweight children. Schools are organizations that are especially pertinent to diabetes prevention. Successful school-based interventions have focused on multiple levels of intervention including environmental change (such as cafeteria food choices), encouraging daily physical activity, classroom instruction by teachers, and family involvement.

    Fear of diabetes complications such as the need for dialysis should not be used to motivate students. Scare tactics are counterproductive (A).

    A letter may increase some parents' awareness about the link between obesity and type 2 diabetes in children; however, some parents may find the letter offensive and the letter is not an intervention to prevent diabetes in the children (C).

    The concern is obesity and development of type 2 diabetes in the children. Screening parents does not provide information about glucose of obese children at risk (D).

99. **B.** The absence of warning signs of impending neuroglycopenia is known as hypoglycemia unawareness. It is a failure of glucose counter-regulation characterized by the diminished glucagon and epinephrine secretion. Severe hypoglycemia is an episode that requires the assistance of another individual to treat. It may or may not occur with warning signs (A). Answers C and D are forms of neuropathies and are therefore not correct.

100. **A.** The correct answer is dehydration. BUN and serum creatinine would be elevated secondary to the dehydration (B). Serum osmolality is increased and the arterial pH is reduced as the result of acidosis (C and D).

101. **B.** Thiazolidinediones is correct. Thiazolidinediones or glitazones increase plasma volume, which may be particularly dangerous for patients with New York Heart Association Class III or IV heart failure. Meglitinides (A), alpha-glucosidase inhibitors (C), and sulfonylureas (D) are all safe to use in patients with heart failure.

Section 4: Answer Key

102. **C.** Rehydration is correct. Adequate rehydration of patients suffering from diabetic ketoacidosis or hyperglycemic hyperosmolar state (HHS) is an essential first step to restore appropriate glucose levels. Correction of electrolyte deficits (B) usually follows rehydration and is accompanied by balanced administration of insulin (A) and glucose replacement (D).

103. **B.** The correct answer is 4 oz of juice. Hypoglycemia is generally treated with 10 to 15 grams of easily absorbed carbohydrate, which should include 4 oz of fruit juice or soda. The addition of sugar is not necessary (C), and 12 oz of soda would equal ~60 grams of carbohydrate (A). Foods high in fat content (such as peanut butter) slow gastric empting and the absorption of carbohydrate (D).

104. **D.** Diabetic ketoacidosis (DKA) is correct. Newly diagnosed patients with type 2 diabetes (A) may have glucose levels as high as 359 mg/dL, but without changes in acid-base status. This presentation is also not consistent with hyperosmolar hyperglycemic state (B), which typically occurs with blood glucose levels higher than 400 mg/dL. Finally, elevated blood glucose levels may contribute to, but are not required to diagnose patients with diabetic nephropathy (C). Diabetic nephropathy is characterized by decreased glomerular filtration (GFR) and proteinuria in a patient with diabetes.

105. **A.** This question is assessing knowledge of appropriate sick-day management for use in prevention of diabetic ketoacidosis (DKA). Early recognition of hyperglycemia and appropriate treatment during illness are essential to prevent DKA. To maintain hydration during illness, 8 oz of fluid per hour is required. Every third hour, the 8 oz of fluid should be a sodium-rich fluid, such as bouillon.

Answers B, C, and D are incorrect. In assessing when to contact the healthcare team during illness, the patient should call if she vomits more than once, if she has diarrhea more than 5 times or for longer than 6 hours, when blood glucose is >300 mg/dL on 2 consecutive measurements that are not responsive to increased insulin and fluids, or when there are moderate or large urine or blood ketones present.

106. **D.** Social support is the correct answer. Having the family present can provide important assessment information and insights into family dynamics.

107. **B.** Flexibility and balance exercises are beneficial, particularly for older adults with diabetes and limited joint mobility, but do not affect glycemia. Balance training can reduce the risk of falls by improving balance and gait. Stretching increases range of motion around joints and flexibility. A, C, and D all improve glycemia.

108. **C.** Insulin causes cells to take in potassium from the plasma is the correct answer. Insulin administration to patients with diabetic ketoacidosis drives potassium into cells from the plasma. To avoid hypokalemia, potassium supplementation may be given with insulin (A and B). Potassium is important for many cellular functions, including insulin release from pancreatic islet cells; however, potassium is not considered an essential cofactor for glucose metabolism (D).

139

Review Guide for the CDE® Exam

109. **D.** Individuals with hyperosmolar hyperglycemic state (HHS) have elevated blood glucose levels >600 mg/dL. HHS occurs primarily in undiagnosed or elderly individuals with type 2 diabetes, eliminating A and B as good choices. Serum osmolality is elevated in both DKA and HHS, and thus C does not support the diagnosis.

110. **D.** Advising him that sildenafil is contraindicated in patients taking nitrates is correct. Type 2 diabetes is a common cause of erectile dysfunction. Although patients with erectile dysfunction may benefit from marriage counseling, there is no evidence that this patient is currently experiencing marital issues (A). All of the phosphodiesterase-5 inhibitors improve erectile dysfunction to similar degrees, so changing from sildenafil to vardenafil would not offer additional benefit (B). Yohimbine improves erectile dysfunction by increasing blood pressure, which would not be useful in this patient with uncontrolled hypertension (C).

111. **D.** Several complications of diabetes, as well as other associated risks, play key roles in the development of diabetic foot problems. These include peripheral vascular disease, neuropathies, improperly fitting shoes, nail abnormalities, visual problems, and lack of self-management skills. Daily foot inspections and proper nail care reduce amputation risk by preventing, or detecting early, any problem areas.

Age is not a factor directly correlated with amputation risk (A).

Wearing shoes without laces could actually increase amputation risk from trauma caused by the loose shoes rubbing the foot and delayed healing secondary to poor blood glucose control (B).

There is not a documented direct correlation between a specific A1C level and amputation risk. However, it is known that elevated A1C increases risk for peripheral vascular disease and neuropathies, which in turn play key roles in the development of diabetic foot problems (C).

112. **B.** B is the correct answer since the A1C goal meets recommended targets and albumin is within the normal range. Answer A is incorrect because the albumin is within the albuminuria range. Answer C is incorrect because the A1C target is too high and albumin is within the albuminuria range. Answer D is an incorrect choice since both goals are too high.

113. **C.** Bargaining is the correct answer. The stages of denial, anger, bargaining, depression, and acceptance described for the process of grief in dying are similar to what an individual facing a new diagnosis of diabetes may feel. MS may or may not go through all of these stages. A, B, and D are incorrect.

114. **A.** Gastroparesis is a diabetic autonomic neuropathy that occurs because of damage to the vagus nerve, which controls the muscles moving food through the digestive tract. Delayed gastric emptying can cause anorexia, nausea, vomiting, early satiety, and postprandial bloating and fullness. It can also produce wide swings between severe

Section 4: Answer Key

hypoglycemia and hyperglycemia. Lifestyle modifications for treatment of gastroparesis include the following:

- Small, frequent meals—which results in less bloating, less early satiety, and lessened possibility of impaired nutritional status
- Reduced fat intake—to produce less delay in gastric emptying
- Reduced fiber intake—which may decrease possibility of bezoar formation
- Soft foods; replacement of solid meals with liquid or blenderized meals—because liquid, but non-hypertonic, meals appear to be digested normally
- Exercise after meals—may increase solid-meal gastric emptying rates
- Adjust insulin doses and timing

There is no benefit in reducing fluid or carbohydrate intake beyond the individual's typical goals (B).

Increased fiber intake is not recommended, but rather reduced fiber intake. Furthermore, exercise is recommended after meals to increase gastric emptying, rather than exercise before meals (C).

Exercising before meals is not indicated (D).

115. **A.** It is not uncommon in type 2 diabetes that microvascular changes precede diagnosis. The current recommendation is examination shortly after diagnosis, making B, C, and D incorrect choices.

116. **A.** A is the correct answer as depression is twice as common in patients with type 1 and type 2 diabetes as the general population. Women with diabetes have 1.6 times the risk of depression compared with their male counterparts (B). Being younger, not being married, and having a low level of education are associated with depression (C). CBT is as effective in treating patients with diabetes as without (D).

117. **B.** The ADA Standards of Care recommend maintaining the usual dietary protein intake because it does not alter glycemia or glomerular filtration rate decline. For patients on dialysis, higher protein intake may be considered.

118. **C.** A blood pressure between 140 and 159 mm Hg systolic and 90 to 99 diastolic is considered stage 1 hypertension. High-normal (A) is defined as an average systolic or diastolic blood pressure ≥90 but <95th percentile for age, sex, and height measure on at least 3 separate days in a child. Prehypertension (B) is 120–139 systolic mm Hg and 80–89 mm Hg diastolic. Stage 2 hypertension (D) is ≥160 systolic and ≥100 diastolic.

119. **B.** Individuals with diabetes are more likely than others to suffer from dental problems and periodontal diseases. Prolonged hyperglycemia and the accumulation of advanced glycation end products in gingival tissue are thought to be primarily responsible for oral complications of diabetes. Periodontal disease is the most prevalent oral complication of diabetes.

While these symptoms (A, C, and D) certainly occur in individuals with diabetes, none of these is the most prevalent oral complication.

Review Guide for the CDE® Exam

120. **B.** Thyroid disorders are the most common autoimmune disorder associated with type 1 diabetes, with an incidence of about 17%. Patients with thyroid autoimmunity may be euthyroid, hypothyroid, or hyperthyroid. Adults with type 1 are also prone to many other autoimmune disorders (A, C, D).

121. **A.** To assess productivity, recording patient name and date of visit will show the number of patients seen each day, and therefore the educator's productivity.

   Behavioral goals are part of the Outcomes Identification step in the process of DSME (B).

   Patient name and telephone number are pertinent data to collect when beginning patient assessment (C).

   Blood pressure and plasma glucose are pertinent data points to collect in the Retinopathy Assessment phase of DSME (D).

122. **D.** Osmotic changes in the lens is correct. Blurred vision that improves and worsens with changes in glucose is likely related to osmotic changes. Detached retina (C), macular degeneration (B), and nonproliferative diabetic retinopathy (A) all represent changes that are constant once they occur.

123. **B.** Current recommendations call for testing all women not previously known to have diabetes using the 75-g oral glucose tolerance test (OGTT) between 24 and 28 weeks of gestation. Although advanced maternal age is a risk factor for GDM, current recommendations are that all pregnant women be screened regardless of age (C). Gestational diabetes mellitus affects about 7% of all pregnancies in the United States (A). Approximately 50% of women have no symptoms or risk factors. Screening only symptomatic women would mean 50% would go undiagnosed (D).

124. **A.** Motivational interviewing is a communication technique consistent with several health behavior change theories. It is a patient-centered approach that aims to identify and resolve ambivalence toward behavior change and stimulate motivation to take action. The four guiding principles of motivational interviewing are expressing empathy, developing discrepancies, rolling with resistance, and supporting self-efficacy.

   The educator empathizes with the patient and offers support. Expressing empathy emphasizes active listening and creating a safe, accepting environment in which the patient can express personal thoughts, feelings, and experiences. The educator's primary role is to identify ambivalence, provide support, and relay facts. Giving advice and direct teaching are avoided. Ultimately, the patient, not the educator, determines the pace and direction of the conversation and makes the decision to work on behavior change.

   The educator attempts to uncover and expose discrepancies between the patient's current behavior and values and future aspirations, assisting the patient to explore negative outcomes related to current behavior, ideally fostering an increased motivation to change (B).

Section 4: Answer Key

This principle encourages the educator to work with the patient when the patient exhibits reluctance to take action, rather than directly confronting the patient. The educator's role is not to coerce but to facilitate the process of developing greater motivation (C).

This principle reinforces the patient's confidence in taking action and making behavior changes. The educator promotes an atmosphere of optimism that helps solidify the patient's beliefs that they can perform the specific tasks they set out to accomplish (D).

125. **B.**   The goal for pregnant women with preexisting diabetes is fasting blood glucose between 60 and 100 mg/dL and an A1C within 1% of the normal range (making C an incorrect answer). In the absence of medical or obstetric complications, pregnant women should accumulate 30 minutes or more of moderate-intensity physical exercise on most if not all days of the week (A). Exercise should be avoided if blood glucose is ≥200 mg/dL (or <60 mg/dL) (D).

126. **C.**   They are increased in late gestation is the correct answer. Insulin resistance tends to increase during gestational diabetes and may require insulin doses similar to those of patients with type 2 diabetes (D). Insulin requirements generally do not decline until after delivery (A and B).

127. **A.**   KL should be screened for gestational diabetes at her first prenatal visit because she has 2 high-risk factors: she is African American and she has a family history for type 2 diabetes. Although women with clinical symptoms should be tested, no symptoms were described in this scenario (B). Average-risk women can be screened between 24 and 28 weeks' gestation and we have already identified that KL is at high risk (C and D).

128. **A.**   This woman should not become pregnant until improved glycemia is achieved, due to the risks of malformations associated with poor metabolic control. The American College of Obstetricians and Gynecologists (ACOG) recommends preconception counseling for women with preexisting diabetes with focus on achieving euglycemia prior to and during the critical period of organogenesis to help prevent anomalies.

While the patient does need to improve her glucose control prior to becoming pregnant, based on current glucose control, insulin is not immediately warranted. The educator would want to explore her current diabetes self-management practices, identify and discuss lifestyle modifications that could be made to achieve tighter control, and then recommend the addition of oral diabetes medications as needed (B).

Recommendations from the ADA Standards of Medical Care state that A1C should be as close to normal as possible (<7%) before conception is attempted (C).

Evidence supports that women with preexisting diabetes can certainly have healthy pregnancies and positive outcomes when achieving optimal glycemic control prior to conception and maintaining euglycemia throughout the pregnancy (D).

143

Review Guide for the CDE® Exam

129. **B.** This is the definition of minimal encouragers. The other 3 choices (A, C, D) are also forms of verbal and nonverbal behaviors generally referred to as active listening skills, but they do not match the definition provided.

130. **C.** Insulin syringe magnifier is correct. This elderly patient is most likely unable to visualize the correct insulin dose due to decreased vision. Changing to a 1/2-mL syringe is inappropriate for this patient because his dose of 52 units will exceed the capacity (A). An insulin pump is inappropriate because this patient is not on multiple daily injections, so the cost would not be justified (B). A jet injector is also inappropriate in this elderly patient due to the large dose and propensity to cause injection site pain (D).

131. **C.** Answer C (honeymoon period) is correct. Many patients with type 1 diabetes experience restored insulin secretion a short time after diagnosis, which decreases the need for exogenous insulin. The dawn phenomenon and Somogyi effect refer to unexpected high fasting blood glucose values (A and B). Insulin that becomes denatured or "spoiled" usually loses it's effectiveness, requiring increased doses to achieve the same effect (D).

132. **C.** The DCCT and the follow-up study EDIC (Epidemiology of Diabetes Interventions and Complications) have shown that intensive treatment and maintenance of glucose concentrations close to the normal range clearly decrease the frequency and severity of the macrovascular and microvascular complications of diabetes. A risk, however, of intensive glycemic control is increased possibility of hypoglycemia.

133. **A.** The impact of pregnancy on retinopathy progression is DF's major concern. According to adult learning theory, adults learn best when they feel the need to know and when it is personally relevant. The other topics are important but can be discussed later (B, C, and D).

134. **C.** Untreated proliferative retinopathy is a contraindication to pregnancy (C). Rapid normalization of blood glucose values (A) and hypertension (D) can cause retinopathy to progress, making them incorrect choices. Regression of retinopathy is common following delivery (B).

135. **A.** Glycemic targets for pregnant women with and without preexisting diabetes are the same. Because fetal complications during pregnancy are related to the extent of hyperglycemia, both the American College of Obstetricians and Gynecologists (ACOG) and the ADA endorse the same targets for all patients. Before meals blood glucose <95 mg/dL, 1-hour postmeal glucose <140 mg/dL, and 2 hours postmeal glucose <120 mg/dL.

136. **A.** Weight loss and at least 150 minutes of exercise weekly is correct. In the Diabetes Prevention Program (DPP), metformin 850 mg twice daily was less effective than lifestyle interventions at preventing diabetes in high-risk individuals (C). Acarbose and rosiglitazone are associated with decreased progression to diabetes; however, neither drug was compared in the DPP study (B and D).

Section 4: Answer Key

137. **D.**   The lifestyle intervention arm of the DPP reduced the risk of developing type 2 diabetes by 58%.

138. **C.**   A weight loss of 5% to 7% of initial body weight has been shown to prevent type 2 diabetes in high-risk individuals.

139. **A.**   According to the 2017 American Association of Clinical Endocrinologists (AACE) guidelines and the 2014 National Association (NLA) recommendations, there is a therapeutic option to set the LDL goal at less than 70 mg/dL for **very high risk** patients—those who have had a recent heart attack, those who have cardiovascular disease combined with either type 1 diabetes or type 2 diabetes, those who have severe or poorly controlled risk factors (such as continued smoking), or those who have metabolic syndrome (a cluster of risk factors associated with obesity that includes high triglycerides and low HDL cholesterol). CC is classified as very high risk because he has cardiovascular disease and diabetes and he smokes.

LDL <100 mg/dL is the treatment goal for **high-risk** individuals, not **very high risk** individuals like CC. Those classified as **high risk** have coronary heart disease (CHD), or disease of the blood vessels to the brain or extremities, or diabetes, or multiple (2 or more) risk factors that give them a greater than 20% chance of having a heart attack within 10 years. CC's risk factors classify him as very high risk (B).

LDL <130 mg/dL is the treatment goal for **moderately high risk** individuals. Moderately high risk individuals have multiple (2 or more) CHD risk factors together with a 10–20% risk for a heart attack within 10 years. CC's risk factors classify him as very high risk (C and D).

140. **C.**   All insulin pumps deliver both basal and bolus insulin. Costs of pumps vary (A). Pump models do not have the same components (B). Pump choice should be based on the needs of the user (D).

141. **D.**   Large doses of aspirin can cause increased basal and stimulated release of insulin.

142. **B.**   For individuals with severe peripheral neuropathy, high-impact weight-bearing activities such as aerobics classes are discouraged. Moderate walking has been shown to reduce the progression of peripheral neuropathy in both type 1 and type 2 diabetes (A). Swimming and chair exercises are non-weight bearing and are therefore also recommended (C, D).

143. **B.**   These (lack of interest in written materials, admission that he does not read much, and excuse of forgotten glasses) are all classic clues that the individual may have low literacy skills.

144. **C.**   Currently, there is insufficient research to support universal use among individuals with diabetes. Major research is under way, however, on complementary and alternative therapies.

Review Guide for the CDE® Exam

Just because a supplement is "natural" doesn't mean it's safe for use. Concerns include potential side effects, drug interactions, variability of products, lack of product standardization, possibility of contamination, delay in using more effective interventions, and additional costs (A).

Complementary therapies can have serious side effects. Ginkgo biloba's side effects include headache, GI upset, bleeding reactions, and seizures if handling or eating the seeds. Bilberry's side effects include mild gastrointestinal distress and skin rashes. Milk thistle's side effects include diarrhea, weakness, sweating, and possible allergic reactions (B).

Natural agents are NOT subject to rigorous government safety and efficacy testing, so they may be potentially more dangerous than conventional forms of medication (D).

145. **C.**   Personal health information must always be stored, analyzed, and reported in a manner that protects the identification of individuals. It is permissible for the educator to contact her patients and advise them of the opportunity so that they can contact the manufacturer directly. Answers A, B, D all violate HIPAA regulations.

146. **C.**   Decrease morning aspart insulin to 4 units is correct. The current dose of aspart insulin is more than that required by her usual carbohydrate intake each morning, which results in frequent hypoglycemia before lunch. Lowering the insulin dose by 10% to 4 units is the most appropriate change. Decreasing the bedtime dose of glargine insulin is inappropriate because it will result in elevated fasting blood glucose values (A). Because glargine insulin doses above 20 units consistently provide a duration of action of at least 24 hours, moving the administration time (B) or splitting the dose (D) will not improve the hypoglycemic frequency.

147. **A.**   Motivational interviewing is a patient-centered approach that aims to identify and resolve ambivalence toward behavior change. Choices B, C, and D are all health behavior change theories and therefore not correct.

148. **D.**   Women with GDM have normal glucose levels early in pregnancy during the period of organogenesis and therefore the risk of giving birth to an infant with a malformation is not increased. Macrosomia, neonatal hypoglycemia, and shoulder dystocia are common complications associated with GDM. Their risk is increased with maternal hyperglycemia.

149. **C.**   While a willingness to learn is important, problem-solving skills, health literacy, and a sound knowledge of diabetes self-care skills and behaviors (A, B, D) are essential for effective pattern management.

150. **B.**   Answers A, C, and D are an appropriate focus/action steps at diagnosis for DSMES. Making a referral for medical nutrition therapy (MNT) is an appropriate action step at diagnosis for a primary care provider or for the clinical care team, as described in the Diabetes Self-management Education and Support in Type 2 Diabetes: A Joint Position Statement of the American Diabetes Association, the American Association of Diabetes Educators, and the Academy of Nutrition and Dietetics.

Section 4: Answer Key

151. **C.**   This question focuses on teaching strategies and the learning experience.

Demonstration, an active form of learning, is the most effective teaching strategy to teach this psychomotor skill. It allows for the educator to demonstrate correct injection technique and for the patient to provide return demonstration for evaluation of technique. This teaching strategy allows the learner to observe, perform, and be evaluated.

Lecture is a passive form of learning and does not allow the educator to evaluate the learner's ability to actually perform insulin injection (A).

Audiovisual aids can add variety to the teaching session and may particularly benefit visual learners; however, they cannot replace demonstration of injection technique with evaluation of return demonstration (B).

Print materials cannot replace in-person education with demonstration and return demonstration for the educator to assess the patient's ability to correctly administer insulin injections (D).

152. **C.**   Ten to fourteen days is correct. Each of the insulin pens and pen cartridges have different stability recommendations. Once opened, the prefilled 70/30 insulin pens are stable at room temperature for 10–14 days. Educators should consult the package insert for specific products before advising patients about stability duration.

153. **C.**   Diabetes educators should avoid any negative connotation to the use of insulin and implications that blame a patient for the progression of their disease. Establishing trust (A), use of motivational interviewing techniques (B), and showing some of the newer options for administration may help alleviate fears about injections (C).

154. **B.**   Chart audit (B) is the correct answer since laboratory values such as A1C would be recorded in the patient's chart. Telephone follow-up and surveys would have to rely on patient self-report of their A1C levels, which might provide inaccurate data, making C and A incorrect choices. If an A1C were to be included as part of the post-program evaluation, it would provide data at one time point only and therefore could not be utilized to detect change, making D incorrect.

155. **B.**   Answer B (Penetration into the target population) is correct. The impact of a program can be determined by evaluating its penetration, implementation, participation, and effectiveness related to the target population. Measuring staff performance (A) is an important internal program measurement, but is not related to population impact. The degree of integration with multiple disciplines (C) or interest in self-care behaviors (D) may be important program goals, but do not determine program impact according to the PIPE model.

156. **B.**   Health status and cost are directly related. Improved health status would reduce the managed care organization's cost. Although enhanced knowledge (A), increased monitoring (C), and healthy eating (D) are important program outcomes, it would be difficult if not impossible to document their cost savings to the organization.

147

Review Guide for the CDE® Exam

157. **B.** Intermediate is correct. An immediate outcome of diabetes self-management education (A), such as knowledge, occurs before the intermediate outcome, such as increased exercise. Post-intermediate outcomes (C) are clinical changes that lead to long-term outcomes (D) as a result of a change in behavior.

158. **D.** Involving family members is critical to support patients as they cope with the psychosocial and behavioral aspects of diabetes self-management. (Source: Diabetes Self-management Education and Support in Type 2 Diabetes: A Joint Position Statement of the American Diabetes Association, the American Association of Diabetes Educators, and the Academy of Nutrition and Dietetics)

159. **D.** Glucose control is considered the leading alterable risk factor associated with the development and progression of diabetes retinopathy. Blood pressure is another important, alterable factor, though it is not considered the primary factor (B). There is less agreement concerning the importance of other risk factors, such as renal disease (A) and age (C).

160. **A.** Standard 7 of the National Standards for Diabetes Self-Management and Support (NSDSMES) states that documentation must occur at every step in the DSME process. Documentation is an ongoing process and not a onetime event (B). Documentation should capture immediate, intermediate, post-intermediate, and long-term outcomes (C). Documentation is protected by HIPAA (D).

161. **C.** Glargine is wearing off early. Glargine insulin serves as a basal insulin to inhibit hepatic glucose output. The ideal basal insulin dose maintains consistent preprandial blood glucose values throughout the day. The correct insulin-to-carbohydrate ratio should maintain peak postprandial blood glucose levels less than 180 mg/dL (A and B). The dawn phenomenon is characterized by elevated fasting glucose levels resulting from inappropriate basal insulin overnight (D).

162. **A.** Breakfast carbohydrate intake is higher on Saturday at 87 grams, versus 30 grams for the weekday breakfast. The higher carbohydrate intake on Saturday correlates with the higher 2-hour postmeal blood glucose on Saturday.

Weekday breakfast total carbohydrate count is **30 grams:**
1/4 cup liquid egg substitute (0 carbs)
2 slices turkey bacon (0 carbs)
1 slice whole wheat toast with margarine (15 carbs)
1/2 cup apple juice (15 carbs)

Saturday breakfast total carbohydrate count is **87 grams:**
2 pancakes (30 carbs)
1/4 cup light syrup (30 carbs)
1/2 banana (15 carbs)
1 cup skim milk (12 carbs)

148

Section 4: Answer Key

163. **C.** Cultural awareness is the recognition of personal prejudices and biases toward other cultures. Other components of a practice model of cultural competence include cultural humility, which is a commitment to ongoing self-evaluation and critiques (A); cultural knowledge, which is an education foundation that incorporates various worldviews of different cultures (B); and cultural desire, which is the commitment to engage in the process of cultural competence (D).

164. **B.** Having a patient actually calculate the carbohydrate content of a typical meal allows the educator to assess the patient's understanding of portion sizes, ability to read and understand food labels, knowledge of correlating carbohydrate content of foods, and math skills.

Asking the patient to keep a food log allows for assessment of typical foods and portion sizes, but does not assess the carbohydrate counting skills. A meal(s) from the food log could be used for the patient to calculate the carbohydrate content of a meal (A).

Asking the patient to list foods high in carbohydrate assesses only their basic knowledge of carbohydrate-rich foods; it does not assess their knowledge of the associated specific carbohydrate content of foods, knowledge of portion sizes, ability to read and understand food labels, or math skills used in calculating the carbohydrate content of a meal (C).

Being able to identify carbohydrate content of foods using the Nutrition Facts panel is just one skill necessary to correctly calculate the carbohydrate content of a meal (D).

165. **C.** Changes in physical activity levels and problem solving are examples of behavior change. Although knowledge and learning are important, they do not ensure behavior change (A). Changes in A1C, lipids, blood pressure, and BMI are examples of improved health status (D). Continuous quality improvement (CQI) is incorrect because it refers to program evaluation (B).

166. **B.** A behavioral goal is based on a planned measurable change in behavior that is expected to have positive health outcomes. The only choice that fits those criteria is answer B. Monitoring blood glucose 3 times a day is a planned measurable change.

167. **A.** In evaluating the log using the ADA Standards of Medical Care in Diabetes, preprandial plasma blood glucose target of 80–130, reported fasting values are in target. Three of the four prelunch values reflect hypoglycemia and one predinner value reflects hypoglycemia, with the other 3 values on the verge of hypoglycemia. Assuming carbohydrate counts are accurate as recorded, the conclusion can be drawn that the breakfast detemir dose should be decreased secondary to the recurrent hypoglycemia.

Decreasing the bedtime detemir dose would allow the blood glucose to rise through the night, causing hyperglycemia in the morning before breakfast (A).

149

Review Guide for the CDE® Exam

Moving the bedtime detemir to before the evening meal would likely increase the risk of insulin stacking with the morning dose, worsening the risk of hypoglycemia (B). Adding predinner aspart would further drive down the blood glucose levels overnight, increasing the risk of nocturnal hypoglycemia as well as the number of daytime episodes. The blood glucose log reflects frequent hypoglycemia—1/3 of the values are in the hypoglycemia range <70 (D).

168. **C.**   Active learning is most appropriate for 6-year-olds. It is important to match teaching strategies to learning styles of the learner, and the other choices fail in this regard.

169. **D.**   Metformin is correct. The immediate release formulation of metformin possesses Food and Drug Administration (FDA) approved product labeling for use in children over age 10. The safety and efficacy of glyburide (A), acarbose (B), and glipizide (C) have not been established in pediatric patients.

170. **C.**   The focus of this question is evaluation of goals and documenting outcomes. Some key areas to consider when evaluating goals include:

1. What is the patient's assessment of the goal?
   • Did the patient feel he achieved the goal?
   • How would he rate his progress?

2. What is the educator's collaborative assessment of the goal?
   • Was the goal appropriate?
   • Was there adequate time to achieve the goal?
   • Did the goal achieve the expected outcome?
   • Did the outcome impact the diabetes treatment plan?
   • Does therapy need to change?

3. What should the next steps be?
   • Should the goal be changed or continued?
   • Should additional goals be added or other goals changed?
   • When will new goals be evaluated?
   • What other changes in the diabetes treatment plan need to occur to support the goal(s)?

The patient's assessment is that exercising 30 minutes 7 days a week is too overwhelming. It appears that the initial goal was too aggressive for this patient. Setting an intermediate goal of working up to 20 minutes 6 or 7 days a week over a longer 3-month period is likely more realistic for this individual (C).

The patient has already relayed that this goal is currently too overwhelming (A).

Maintaining the patient's current activity level does not further work him toward a long-term goal of 30 minutes 7 days a week (B).

SECTION 4: ANSWER KEY

150

Section 4: Answer Key

There is no need to discontinue exercise altogether. At this point, some is better than none, and setting an intermediate goal assists the patient in working toward a long-term goal of 30 minutes 7 days a week (D).

171. **D.**   It is important to match education materials to literacy skills of the patient. Answer A is incorrect because it is still appropriate to provide written materials as long as they are at the correct reading level. Although it is important to include the family in the teaching, the wife does not have to attend all the classes (B). There is no evidence provided suggestive of a cognitive deficit (C).

172. **D.**   Check his blood glucose and call emergency services if it is normal is correct. The patient's symptoms and presentation history of recent exertion are not consistent with hyperglycemia (B). Patients with type 2 diabetes are at significantly increased risk of cardiovascular disease. Because symptoms of hypoglycemia and myocardial infarction overlap, the correct intervention sequence begins with ruling out hypoglycemia by testing the patient's blood glucose. Providing sources of carbohydrate (A and C) before testing the blood glucose makes it impossible to correctly identify hypoglycemia as the cause.

173. **B.**   Lancing devices, lancets, or meters should not be shared (unless the meters are cleaned and disinfected after each use) (D). Cleaning the endcap does not eliminate the risk of blood-borne pathogen transmission (B). Cleaning and disinfecting instructions are included in the meter owner's manual (A). Sharps containers or other containers approved by the state may be used to dispose of lancets or other sharps (C). Where blood glucose monitoring is performed by someone other than the patient, such as in a long-term care facility, clinic, or school, single use, auto-disabling lancets must be used.

174. **D.**   Aspirin is correct. Patients with type 2 diabetes are at significantly increased risk of myocardial infarction. This patient with established cardiovascular disease would benefit most by adding aspirin to his regimen. Cinnamon (A), chromium picolinate (B), and ginseng (C) may improve glucose tolerance; however, data to support their use are limited.

175. **A.**   Although lack of concentration is consistent with depression, sweating and restlessness are not (B). Elevated blood glucose levels would be expected with the flu (C). There is no evidence to suggest fear of social situations (D).

176. **B.**   An ophthalmologist should perform a dilated examination annually is correct. Patients with diabetes should receive annual dilated eye examinations to ensure healthy vision. Less frequent screening may be appropriate for patients with good glycemic control following one or more normal eye examinations. Although additional screening by endocrinologists (A and D) or optometrists (C) may be useful, dilation of the eye is necessary to identify presence of blood retinal damage in the lateral portions of the eye. Furthermore, only ophthalmologists can initiate corrective therapy if retinal damage is identified.

151

Review Guide for the CDE® Exam

177. **A.** Fetal complications associated with maternal hyperglycemia include congenital malformations, neonatal hypoglycemia, macrosomia, stillbirth, respiratory distress, hyperbilirubinemia, hypocalcemia, and polycythemia. The American College of Obstetricians and Gynecologists (ACOG) recommends preconception counseling for women with preexisting diabetes, with focus on achieving euglycemia prior to and during the critical period of organogenesis to help prevent anomalies.

Congenital anomalies occur during organogenesis, the first 8 weeks of gestation. Therefore, it is critical for women with preexisting diabetes to receive preconception care in order to achieve euglyemia prior to conception.

Preconception care to achieve euglycemia is beneficial for ALL women with preexisting diabetes (B).

There is no correlation between preconception care and increased fertility (C).

Preconception care is just that, care prior to conception in order to achieve euglycemia to help prevent anomalies (D).

178. **C.** According to the National Kidney Foundation, this patient has Stage 3 chronic kidney disease as evidenced by the presence of albumin in the urine and moderately decreased eGFR.

179. **B.** Feeling down and depressed, difficulty falling asleep, and difficulty concentrating are clues to the educator that TK may be depressed. Depression is twice as common in individuals with diabetes. Diabetes educators play a key role in screening their patients for depression. TK reveals clues that she may be depressed. Referral to a mental health professional for further evaluation is warranted.

TK reveals symptoms of depression, so further evaluation and treatment are currently warranted. Identifying and addressing depression is important in order to facilitate the patient's adherence to self-care plans (A).

The symptoms are consistent with depression and not necessarily stress. She would gain most benefit from referral to a mental health professional that could assess need for and provide psychotherapy and pharmacotherapy (C).

Providing education does not address or resolve the underlying problem (D).

180. **C.** Refer him and his wife to a marriage counselor is correct. The marital problems of this patient are long-standing and are interfering with his diabetes management. The most appropriate action is to refer him and his wife to counseling. Refocusing the conversation (A) or rescheduling the appointment (B) inappropriately dismisses this patient's primary concern. The patient's psychological changes are secondary to an identifiable cause and do not likely require medication therapy at this time (D).

Section 4: Answer Key

181. **D.** It is common for parents to be overwhelmed with fears and the stress of learning new skills and managing new responsibilities associated with having a child with newly diagnosed diabetes. The diabetes educator and healthcare team should be instrumental in assisting families dealing with these issues. Answer choices A, B, and C are acceptable to say to or provide to the parents, but Answer D is the best choice because it offers the parents concrete assistance if they are facing challenges managing their child's diabetes.

182. **B.** The main concerns are EW's elevated blood pressure and total cholesterol. Otherwise, EW's A1C indicates blood glucose control within target. EW has a normal weight BMI. The DASH eating plan is an acronym for Dietary Approaches to Stop Hypertension. It emphasizes a diet high in fruits, vegetables, and low-fat dairy foods and is low in total fat, saturated fat, and cholesterol. Not only would the DASH eating plan help improve EW's blood pressure, the reduction in fat and cholesterol would benefit EW's cholesterol.

    A low carbohydrate diet would primarily impact blood glucose control, rather than directly impacting blood pressure and lipids (A). A low-fat diet alone would not address EW's hypertension, although it could positively impact lipids (C). Carbohydrate counting in an otherwise unrestricted diet would primarily impact blood glucose, not blood pressure and lipids (D).

183. **C.** A chart audit would be the best tool for collecting this type of data. Time studies (A) are best used to collect concurrent information about the time needed to complete a process. Checklists (B) are useful for gathering concurrent information during a study. Surveys (D) are best used for questioning individuals. Self-report, however, would not be as reliable as a chart audit.

184. **D.** Individuals interested in using pump therapy need to master a variety of skills as a prerequisite to initiation of insulin pump therapy. These skills include:

    • Frequent blood glucose monitoring
    • Carbohydrate counting
    • Calculating bolus insulin
    • Problem solving through interpretation of blood glucose patterns
    • Insulin adjustment

    Carbohydrate counting is a skill that an individual must master prior to using an insulin pump. The ability to accurately count carbohydrates is essential in order to accurately calculate bolus insulin.

    While an exercise plan is a key component of the diabetes self-management plan, the exercise plan is not a prerequisite for insulin pump therapy (A).

153

Review Guide for the CDE® Exam

The ability to carbohydrate count, rather than calorie count, is the critical prerequisite skill for pump therapy (B).

A formal psychological evaluation is not indicated prior to the initiation of pump therapy. The educator should be able to assess an individual's interest, motivation, and ability to use pump therapy (C).

185. **D.** Community meal program is correct. The most likely cause of this patient's weight loss and hypoglycemia is related to her inability to purchase and prepare her food. There is no indication of financial barriers or nutritional deficits that could be resolved by a financial counselor (C) or dietitian (A). Glipizide is appropriate for this patient as indicated by the fact that she is not gaining weight and only experiences occasional hypoglycemia (B), so a pharmacist intervention is also unlikely to resolve her issues.

186. **B.** Individuals with type 2 diabetes should have a comprehensive dilated eye examination annually. Since the patient has not had an eye examination in 5 years it is clearly the only correct choice.

187. **C.** A diagnosis of diabetes can be made when symptoms of hyperglycemia are present and a casual plasma glucose is ≥200 mg/dL or an A1C is >6.5%. This patient's fasting glucose is 498 mg/dL and A1C is 13.4%—both are profoundly elevated. He is exhibiting classic symptoms of hyperglycemia—polydipsia, polyuria, rapid and unplanned weight loss, and fatigue. The key indicator of a likely diagnosis of type 2 diabetes, rather than type 1 diabetes, is the absence of serum ketones. Individuals with type 1 diabetes typically present with serum ketones (due to absolute insulin deficiency).

Answer A is incorrect based on the above explanation.

Serum ketones were negative. Serum ketones must be positive to consider a diagnosis of diabetic ketoacidosis (DKA). When ketone accumulation is excessive, blood becomes too acidic to support life. DKA can be mild, moderate, or severe, depending on parameters of blood glucose levels, acidity, and ketone formation (B).

Impaired fasting glucose is classified as fasting glucose of 100–125 mg/dL, whereas this patient's fasting glucose is 498 mg/dL (D).

188. **C.** Glargine insulin is correct. This patient has significant hyperglycemia as evidenced by his A1C and fasting blood glucose. Pioglitazone (A), acarbose (B), and exenatide (D) are each only capable of reducing A1C by 1% to 1.5%; however, this patient needs significantly greater glucose lowering to reach his goal of less than 7%. As monotherapy, only insulin will be able to help him reach his glycemic goal.

189. **B.** The patient clearly needs treatment for his diabetes (he is symptomatic and has a very elevated A1C) and has no insurance. Nothing in the scenario indicates that he is homebound or having mental health issues or cardiac problems, making the other choices incorrect.

154

Section 4: Answer Key

190. **A.** In a patient-centered approach, collaboration and effective communication are considered the route to patient engagement. This approach includes such skills as eliciting emotions, perceptions, and knowledge through active and reflective listening, asking open-ended questions, exploring the desire to learn or change, and supporting self-efficacy.

191. **C.** Surveys can be used to measure both behavior change and satisfaction. Process data are best collected using chart/file audits or checklists (A). Lab data are best collected using chart/file audits (B). Scheduling issues are best handled via a time study (D).

192. **B.** The transtheoretical model of behavior change focuses on an individual's readiness to make a behavior change and is marked by 6 distinct stages: Precontemplation, Contemplation, Preparation, Action, Maintenance, and Termination. It views behavior change as an ongoing process rather than a specific outcome. During the process the individual will have different levels of motivation to change.

In the Contemplation stage, the individual is aware of the problem (ie, risks of hyperglycemia in pregnancy) and intends to change her behavior (ie, improved diabetes self-management), knows the benefits associated with the health behavior change (ie, euglycemia and health baby), and is acutely aware of the drawbacks (ie, hyperglycemia with potential for fetal anomalies/complications). In the Contemplation stage the individual can be in a state of ambivalence.

In the Precontemplation stage, the individual is NOT aware of the problem and has NO intentions of changing her health behavior. This patient IS aware of the problem and HAS intentions of changing her behavior (A).

In the Preparation stage the individual makes plans that will facilitate the health behavior change. This individual has not made specific plans to achieve euglycemia (C).

In the Maintenance stage the individual demonstrates the ability to sustain behavior, which this individual has not yet achieved (D).

193. **D.** Sulfonylureas improve insulin secretion, (A) Thiazolidnediones increase insulin sensitivity, (B) and DPP-4 inhibitors (C) work within the gut to inhibit the breakdown of GLP-1, an incretin hormone.

194. **C.** Dietary Reference Intake (DRI) for carbohydrate for pregnant women is a minimum of 175 grams per day. For nonpregnant women, the recommendation is 130 grams per day (A).

195. **A.** A lack of finances can be a powerful barrier to diabetes self-management education (DSME). Cultural beliefs (B), health beliefs (C), and literacy (D) can also be barriers. However, the fact that the individual has no insurance, has high medical bills, and becomes tearful at the mention of an additional purchase clearly indicates finances need to be assessed by the educator.

SECTION 4: ANSWER KEY

Review Guide for the CDE® Exam

196. **C.** Teenager demonstration of injection technique is correct. Patients should be empowered to perform self-care behaviors whenever possible. Teenagers are generally able to self-inject insulin without parent supervision (A and B). Direct observation rather than verbal description is the most appropriate method to assess injection technique by the patient (D).

197. **B.** The American Diabetes Association (ADA) has set this goal (<7%).

198. **A.** Chronic care model is correct. Social cognitive theory (B) is a model based on the belief that people learn by observing others. The health belief model (C) employs patient perceptions of disease susceptibility, illness severity, barriers to health, and benefits to predict health behaviors. The theory of reasoned action (D) proposes that behavior change results from the interaction between attitude, subjective norms, and behavior intention.

199. **C.** It is important to teach family members or other support persons how to help the individuals with diabetes self-manage their disease. Answer C is the only choice that actively involves the daughter.

200. **C.** 180 mg/dL is correct. Pregnant women and individuals without diabetes should expect 1-hour and 2-hour postprandial capillary glucose levels to remain less than 140 mg/dL and 120 mg/dL respectively (A and B). Plasma glucose levels above 200 mg/dL are not appropriate for any patient (D).

Exam 2

1. **C.** Studies have shown that the greatest predictor of A1C lowering for all age groups using CGM was frequency of sensor use, which was highest in those aged 25 and older and lower in younger age groups (D). A1C lowering has not been associated with the frequency of device calibration (A). Studies have shown that CGM users spend less time in hypo- and hyperglycemia if they respond to the alarms and alerts, but it is not related to the actual alarm settings (B).

2. **A.** Although the other choices (B, C, D) do play a pathologic role in the causation of type 1 diabetes, GAD has been shown to be the best predictor for the future development of type 1 diabetes.

3. **C.** Latent autoimmune diabetes of adults (LADA) is the correct answer (C). Patients with LADA are typically less than 40 years old and often misdiagnosed with type 2 diabetes at presentation (B). Because these patients initially respond to oral agents and do not require insulin, they are usually not diagnosed with type 1 diabetes (A). However, these patients usually progress to insulin requirement over a period of several months, leading some experts to consider LADA related to type 1 diabetes. This patient would not be diagnosed with gestational diabetes because she is not pregnant (D).

4. **D.** The pathophysiologic stages in the development of type 1 diabetes include a genetic predisposition (stage 1), an environmental trigger (stage 2), and active autoimmunity

156

Section 4: Answer Key

(stage 3), making the first 3 choices correct. Peripheral insulin resistance (D) is a defect seen in type 2 diabetes.

5. **A.**   Although 1–2 drinks/day may reduce the risk of cardiovascular (CV) disease, non-drinkers should not be advised to start drinking alcoholic beverages or to drink more often (B). Carbohydrates should not be omitted when drinking alcoholic beverages for persons taking insulin due to the risk of hypoglycemia (C). Studies show that light to moderate drinking reduces blood pressure in both women and men, but chronic, excessive drinking (ie, more than 3 drinks/day) appears to increase blood pressure.

6. **B.**   Telephone the pharmacy to verify the last refill date (B) is correct. The provider suspects poor adherence with this patient, but needs to confirm with additional information. Confronting the patient will likely only result in denial (A). Additional questioning of the patient may reveal intolerable side effects, but changing the metformin formulation is premature at this point (C). Review of the self-monitored blood glucose (SMBG) log is important, but will not confirm the suspected poor adherence (D).

7. **B.**   The amount of carbohydrate and fat should be individualized based on a number of factors. Research does not support an ideal percentage of carbohydrate, protein, or fat intake for persons with diabetes (A, C, D).

8. **C.**   Ask permission from the patient to include her mother in the visit (C) is correct. Although cognitive deficits are noted during the visit, patient trust and confidentiality should be maintained unless clear danger is identified (D). Role-playing will likely not be useful in this patient with thought disorganization (B). Objective data are useful, but alone will not provide sufficient information to accurately evaluate drug therapy (A).

9. **B.**   The ADA Standards of Care recommend A1C testing at least twice yearly in patients who are meeting their glycemic targets. Patients on insulin who have recently changed therapy and those who are not meeting their glycemic targets should have an A1C test performed quarterly.

10. **B.**   The Dietary Approaches to Stop Hypertension (DASH) diet emphasizes fruits, vegetables, low-fat dairy products, whole grains, poultry, fish, and nuts and is reduced in saturated fat, sweets, and sugar-containing beverages. The DASH diet has been shown to lower blood pressure due to the total eating pattern, including the reduction in sodium and the benefits of potassium and other nutrients. It is not recommended to start drinking alcoholic beverages for the cardiovascular benefits if one is currently not drinking, especially in individuals with hypertriglyceridemia (A). Table salt, sea salt, and kosher salt contain very similar amounts of sodium chloride, so using one over the other will not affect AE's blood pressure; in addition, the majority of AE's sodium intake appears to be from eating in restaurants and eating processed foods (C). Given AE's time constraints and her long commute to work, encouraging walking at lunchtime would likely work better in her schedule than going to a gym 5 days/week; resistance training has not consistently been shown to improve blood pressure (D).

157

Review Guide for the CDE® Exam

11. **D.** Basic carb counting can often improve glycemia in type 2 diabetes very quickly. Taking her lunch and eating dinner at home more frequently can significantly reduce her sodium intake and calories, thereby reducing her blood pressure and helping with weight loss goals. Counting both calories and carbs would be more time-consuming and would not focus on her hypertension (A). Learning to choose healthier options at a fast-food restaurant would take more time and effort, and an exchange-type diet is a more complex regimen than needed for AE at this time (B). She will consume less saturated fats and salt (C) by eating out less frequently.

12. **B.** A combination of following the DASH dietary plan and reducing sodium has been shown to be more effective at reducing blood pressure than sodium reduction alone. Reducing the amount of salt one uses at the table generally does not have as much impact as reducing the number of processed foods consumed (A). It is estimated that 77% of sodium in the typical American diet comes from processed foods (C). The current recommendations by the American Diabetes Association (ADA) are to reduce sodium to less than 2,300 mg/day for individuals with diabetes and that further reduction should be individualized (D).

13. **A.** Intensive lifestyle modifications (A) is correct. The Diabetes Prevention Program (DPP) enrolled patients at high risk to develop diabetes and randomized them to usual care, intensive lifestyle modification, or metformin. The group that engaged in intensive lifestyle modifications, including loss of 7% body weight and 150 minutes of exercise each week, was least likely to develop diabetes.

14. **B.** Inability to pay for insulin (B). Unfortunately, insulin is still quite expensive compared with the oral agents for diabetes. Transportation is often a significant issue for homeless patients, but this patient rides his bicycle for transportation (A). Many patients eat only 1 meal per day, which can be easily accommodated with appropriate insulin scheduling. Because this patient eats his large meal in the evening, a high blood glucose level in the afternoon is not affected by that meal (C). Insulin does adhere to some plastic containers, but not enough to elicit a sudden lack of efficacy (D).

15. **C.** Liraglutide and other GLP-1 receptor agonists improve glycemic control in four (4) ways: (1) increased insulin secretion from beta-cells in a glucose-dependent manner; (2) decreased glucagon release from alpha-cells (A); (3) decreased gastric emptying (D); and (4) increased centrally mediated satiety (B).

16. **C.** Currently, there is no consistent evidence linking blood pressure reduction with resistance training. There is strong evidence to show that weight loss reduces blood pressure even if the degree of weight loss is small. The Seventh Report of the Joint National Committee on Prevention, Detection, Evaluation and Treatment of High Blood Pressure (JNC7) summary reports that a 5- to 10-mm Hg reduction in systolic blood pressure is possible per 10 kg of weight loss (A). Reducing sodium intake by at least 1,000 mg/day lowers blood pressure, even if the desired daily sodium intake is not yet achieved (B). Following a dietary plan similar to the DASH eating plan

SECTION 4: ANSWER KEY

158

Section 4: Answer Key

that emphasizes intake of vegetables, fruits, and whole grains; includes low-fat dairy products, poultry, fish, legumes, and nuts; and limits intake of sweets, sugar-sweetened beverages, and red meats has been shown to lower blood pressure in individuals with hypertension (D).

17. **C.** Omega-3 fatty acids are associated with a reduction of triglycerides, but not LDL-cholesterol. Weight loss, substituting unsaturated fats for saturated fats, and consumption of foods fortified with plant sterols and stanols have all been shown to reduce LDL-cholesterol.

18. **D.** Irbesartan (D) is correct. Patients with renal artery stenosis may display a rise in serum creatinine following administration of an angiotensin-converting enzyme (ACE) inhibitor or angiotensin receptor blocker (ARB). Although ACE and ARB drugs decrease glomerular pressure by vasodilating the efferent arteriole, patients with renal artery stenosis are unable to provide compensatory constriction of the afferent arteriole to maintain a minimum glomerular pressure. The result is poor filtration of creatinine and elevation in the plasma. None of the other options (A or B) affect blood flow through the kidney, though elimination of metformin (C) depends on good kidney function.

19. **B.** Walk 150 minutes per week (B) is correct. African Americans are at high risk of developing diabetes and the church members should be encouraged to make positive behavior changes (D). The Diabetes Prevention Program (DPP) enrolled patients at high risk to develop diabetes and randomized them to usual care, intensive lifestyle modification, or metformin. The group that engaged in intensive lifestyle modifications, including loss of 7% body weight and 150 minutes of exercise each week, was least likely to develop diabetes. Fad diets such as frequent fasting (A) and focus on specific foods (C) are not sustainable and poorly supported by the literature.

20. **A.** A is the correct answer, indicating clear evidence from well-conducted, generalizable randomized controlled trials. Levels B and C indicate supportive evidence from cohort studies of poorly controlled or uncontrolled studies respectively. Level E indicates expert consensus or clinical experience.

21. **C.** Switch from fruit juice to water to avoid excess calories (C) is correct. Patients who gain weight often forget to count calories contained in their drink choices. This patient increased her intake of calories by switching to fruit juice. A better choice would be to consume fresh fruits and drink water (B). Because of the calorie content in fried foods, all patients interested in losing weight should avoid these choices (D). Although exercise is important for overall health, the greatest effect on weight comes from dietary choices and calorie limits, not from increasing exercise (A).

22. **D.** Middle-of-the-night hypoglycemia is the most likely cause of her symptoms. Taking her second injection before dinner means that the intermediate-acting insulin (in the 70/30 combination) is peaking in the middle of the night. Although many patients will be awaken by hypoglycemia, some will not. For those who don't wake up with a headache, increased nightmares and night sweats are common symptoms.

Review Guide for the CDE® Exam

23. **D.** Vitamin B12 is found in meat, poultry, fish, and dairy products and is fortified in foods such as breakfast cereals, nondairy milks, soy protein foods, and some margarines. Vegans are strongly encouraged to consume foods fortified with Vitamin B12 daily or to take a supplement. Vitamin C is plentiful in fruits and vegetables (A). Protein is found in beans, peas, lentils, and soybeans and their products, as well as in nuts and nut butters, and seeds (B). Niacin is found in many foods in a vegan diet, including vegetables, grains, nuts, fortified breads, and cereals (C).

24. **C.** Fear of nocturnal hypoglycemia (C) is correct. Patients who experience severe hypoglycemia are often fearful of future events. This fear may result in withholding insulin, especially at bedtime, which results in elevated fasting glucose and A1C levels. Patients with type 1 diabetes may have insulin antibodies, but exogenous insulin administration does not affect antibody levels (A) or insulin resistance (D). This patient already takes 4 injections daily, so fear of multiple injections does not appear to be an issue (B).

25. **A.** Because of the general health benefits of fiber, the American Diabetes Association (ADA) recommends the same guidelines for individuals with diabetes as for the general public, 14 g/1,000 kcals daily or about 25 grams per day for women and 38 grams per day for men.

26. **C.** Valsartan (C) is correct. Progression of microvascular complications depends on effective control of blood glucose and blood pressure. This patient's blood pressure remains above goal on hydrochlorothiazide and would benefit from an angiotensin receptor blocker. Gabapentin is useful to treat patients with peripheral neuropathic pain but does not prevent the complication (A). Simvastatin (B) and aspirin (D) are useful to avoid macrovascular disease.

27. **B.** An A1C of 8.0% corresponds to a mean glucose of 183 mg/dL. Answer A represents an A1C of 7%, answer C represents an A1C of 9%, and answer D corresponds to an A1C of 10%.

28. **A.** Current research suggests that fiber intake to improve glycemic control requires >50 g fiber per day (A). Most studies show that total dietary fiber, especially from natural food sources, seems to have a beneficial effect on serum cholesterol levels and other cardiovascular (CVD) risk factors such as blood pressure (B). The usual amount of dietary fiber consumption in the United States is only about 15 grams per day (C). Fiber has not been shown to lower HDL cholesterol (D).

29. **A.** Aspirin 81 mg daily (A) is correct. This patient with coronary artery disease and diabetes is at high risk of future coronary events and would benefit from aspirin therapy. Inhibition of platelet aggregation requires only small doses of aspirin, 75 to 160 mg daily; higher aspirin doses inhibit prostaglandins and relieve pain (B). Clopidogrel is useful in those patients who do not tolerate aspirin, but is considered second line (C). Warfarin inhibits Vitamin K–dependent clotting factors, but is not useful in prevention of coronary artery disease (D).

SECTION 4: ANSWER KEY

160

Section 4: Answer Key

30. **A.** The amount of saturated fat, cholesterol, and *trans* fat recommended for individuals with diabetes is the same as for the general population. There is no evidence to suggest that there is an ideal amount of total fat for all people with diabetes; therefore, goals should be individualized (B). Saturated fat should be limited to <10% (B, C). Cholesterol should be limited to <300 mg/d (C, D) and *trans* fat limited as much as possible.

31. **B.** Waist circumference >35 inches (B) is correct. Metabolic syndrome is a constellation of metabolic abnormalities that place patients at high risk of cardiovascular disease. Diagnosis of metabolic syndrome is made in patients possessing any 3 of the following 5 criteria: large waist circumference (>35 inches for women, >40 inches for men); fasting triglyceride level >150 mg/dL; low HDL cholesterol (<50 mg/dL for women, <40 mg/dL for men); fasting blood glucose >100 mg/dL; blood pressure >135/85 mm Hg or on treatment.

32. **A.** The ADA Standards of Care recommend that individuals with longer duration of diabetes (C) and known history of severe hypoglycemia (D) may benefit from less, not more, aggressive targets. Limited resources and a lack of social support are also barriers to intensive therapy (B).

33. **D.** The DASH eating plan includes carbohydrate from low-fat dairy, fruits, vegetables, whole grains, and beans and legumes (A and B). It places more emphasis on fish and poultry and less on red meat (C).

34. **D.** Decreased release of incretins (D) is correct. Patients with type 2 diabetes have inappropriately high levels of glucagon release (C) and subsequent gluconeogenesis (A). Diabetes is also characterized by insulin resistance and progressive beta cell destruction (B).

35. **D.** The American Diabetes Association (ADA) recommends 2 or more servings of fish per week, especially fatty fish such as salmon, mackerel, and herring, as a good source of omega-3 fatty acids. Evidence does not support recommending routine use of omega-3 supplements to prevent cardiovascular events (A). Wild-caught fish does not contain larger amounts of omega-3 than farm-raised fish and therefore is not specifically recommended (B). Alfalfa sprouts do not contain omega-3s; there is limited evidence currently showing benefits of consuming chia seeds, and flaxseed oil contains a plant-based omega-3, which is much less effective than marine omega-3s (C).

36. **D.** All are known factors that contribute to glucose variability.

37. **B.** Encourage her to consult with a local podiatrist (B) is correct. This patient has peripheral neuropathy and a history of lower extremity amputation, placing her at high amputation risk. Rubbing alcohol may dry out her skin, allowing bacteria to invade the tissue (A). Over-the-counter corn removers (C) and home surgery (D) are not good choices for this patient, who may not realize the degree of damage inflicted by these interventions.

Review Guide for the CDE® Exam

38. **D.** Patients using 6-mm or longer needles should pinch a skinfold for the medication to reach its intended absorption site. Four- or 5-mm needles can be used by all, including lean and obese adults as well as lean and obese children (B). In children or frail adults, it is recommended that the needle be inserted at a 45 degree angle (C).

39. **B.** Dulaglutide is correct. Most GLP-1 receptor agonists promote 2.5 kg weight loss over 6 months of use. Thiazolidinediones (A) mobilize visceral fat and promote deposition in the peripheral tissue. Insulin secretagogues such as sulfonylureas (C) and meglitinides (D) increase circulating insulin levels resulting in weight gain.

40. **B.** The nutrition label contains a lot of information that can be confusing to many people. The minimal amount of information needed to count carbohydrate would be the serving size and the total carbohydrate. Sugars and sugar alcohols represent only part of the carbohydrate (A, C, D).

41. **C.** Count Your Carbs: Getting Started is the best option for MA at this time, as it is the simplest approach listed that focuses primarily on carbohydrates and provides diabetes-specific information. The Mediterranean and DASH eating plans are healthy eating plans that address all food groups (A, D). Choose Your Foods: Food Lists for Diabetes (previously referred to as Exchange Lists) can be used for carbohydrate counting, but is a more complex approach (B).

42. **C.** Each carbohydrate choice (or serving) is equal to 15 grams of carbohydrate.

43. **B.** Insulin resistance (B) is correct. Acanthosis nigricans, or hyperpigmentation around the neck or axillary region, is associated with insulin resistance. It is unrelated to hygiene (A) or genetics per se (C). Drugs that worsen insulin resistance, such as niacin or hydrochlorothiazide, may induce acanthosis nigricans; however, metformin improves insulin resistance and does not cause this adverse effect (D).

44. **C.** Control solution is used to determine if strips are reading in the correct range as indicated on the vial of strips. Leaving the cap off the vial of strips exposes the strips to humidity and can result in deterioration of the strips and incorrect readings.

45. **C.** In addition, the Mediterranean diet is characterized by moderate alcohol consumption; a high consumption of legumes, fruits, vegetables, and nonrefined cereals; a low consumption of meat and meat products; and a moderate consumption of mild and dairy products.

46. **C.** Pioglitazone (C) is correct. Thiazolidinediones (TZDs) activate PPAR-gamma receptors that promote deposition of free fatty acids into subcutaneous adipose tissue. Deposition of free fatty acids reduces circulating plasma levels, leading to improved insulin resistance, but also results in weight gain. Pramlintide (A) and saxagliptin (C) are weight neutral, and exenatide (B) promotes weight loss.

Section 4: Answer Key

47. **C.** Considering that LL eats at restaurants frequently and that she is very inactive, SMBG may encourage LL to make changes in her food choices when she observes the effect of large portion sizes from restaurants and the effect of physical activity, such as walking, on glucose levels. She is close to the maximum dosage of metformin with an A1C of 7.5% (A). Metformin alone does not generally promote hypoglycemia (B). Considering her A1C and her BMI, insulin would not likely be considered at this point.

48. **D.** Liraglutide (D) is correct. GLP-1 agonists slow gastrointestinal motility and promote satiety centrally resulting in weight loss of up to 5 lbs per year. Sulfonylureas (glyburide, A) and insulin (detemir, B) tend to promote weight gain in patients who continue to consume excess calories after starting these agents. Saxagliptin (C) and other DPP-4 inhibitors are considered weight neutral.

49. **D.** Low albumin does not affect the A1C results. Hemoglobinopathies such as sickle cell anemia (A), iron deficiency (B), and iron supplementation (C) can result in false high or false low A1C results, depending on the methodology used.

50. **D.** In individuals with both prediabetes and diabetes, triglycerides are generally elevated, HDL is low, and LDL may be either increased, borderline, or normal.

51. **D.** Health literacy (D) is correct. This patient is well educated, as evidenced by his profession as a chemistry professor. Although the ability to read (literacy, B) and work with numbers (numeracy, A) is important, education level (C) does not necessarily translate into functional health literacy.

52. **B.** Comparing the 90-day meter average with the A1C that also reflects an average glycemia over a 2–3 month period would be recommended. Failing to check BG results at variable times (A), meter inaccuracy (C), and using an incorrect technique such as using outdated strips or not getting an adequate blood sample (D) could all result in a discrepancy with the A1C result.

53. **A.** Dapagliflozin (A) is correct. Combination of an SGLT2 inhibitor (dapagliflozin) may promote weight loss with low hypoglycemia risk in this active patient. Glipizide (B) and glargine (D) may increase the risk of hypoglycemia and weight gain due to the presence of excess plasma insulin. Thiazolidinediones (TZDs), like pioglitazone (C), activate PPAR-gamma receptors that promote deposition of free fatty acids into subcutaneous adipose tissue. Deposition of free fatty acids reduces circulating plasma levels, leading to improved insulin resistance, but also results in weight gain.

54. **A.** Insulin decreases while glucagon, epinephrine, norepinephrine, growth hormone, and cortisol all increase in response to acute physical activity.

55. **B.** Temperatures in a vehicle parked in the sun in temperatures over 80 degrees Fahrenheit can reach 120–140 degrees Fahrenheit, according to the Centers for Disease Control and Prevention (CDC). Storing strips at temperatures and humidity outside the recommended range can shorten the life of the strips. Different brands of glucose strips

163

Review Guide for the CDE® Exam

may underestimate or overestimate the glucose value, and the meter is usually unable to detect a problem with the bad strip. Because JG's incorrect readings are sporadic—perhaps occurring during the hotter season—it is less likely that incorrect results would be due to an inaccurate meter, expired strips, or calibration.

56. **B.** Although the actual need will vary from person to person, the general guideline is 0 to 10 grams for every 30 minutes of mild activity, 5 to 10 grams for every 15 minutes of moderate activity, and 0 to 15 grams for every 15 minutes of high-intensity aerobic physical activity.

57. **D.** Canagliflozin side effect (D) is correct. Canagliflozin, an SGLT2 inhibitor, promotes glucose excretion in the urine, which lowers plasma glucose levels but also increases the risk of urinary tract infections. This patient has excellent glycemic control (A) that is well below the threshold for passive glucose disposal in the urine (plasma glucose >180 mg/dL). Metformin is eliminated via the kidneys but is not associated with increased risk of urinary tract infections (B). Although caffeine intake (C) may increase urination, it also is not associated with the other symptoms that this patient reports (urgency, dysuria).

58. **C.** Studies in women with gestational diabetes have shown that postprandial testing is more closely associated with a lower incidence of complications. The American Diabetes Association (ADA) and the American College of Obstetricians and Gynecologists (ACOG) recommend postmeal testing.

59. **D.** Bradycardia (D) is correct. Hypoglycemia is characterized by blood glucose levels less than 70 mg/dL. Symptoms of hypoglycemia include the following: hunger (A), tiredness or weakness (C), tachycardia, sweating, shakiness, agitation (B), nervousness, and unclear thinking.

60. **B.** Due to the potential lag in change in glucose levels when glucose is changing rapidly, AST should only be used when glucose levels are relatively stable if the person is at risk for hypoglycemia.

61. **C.** Consume tablets with 15 to 20 g of glucose (C) is correct. This patient presents with mild hypoglycemia (blood glucose <70 mg/dL characterized by sweating, shaking, hunger, feelings of anxiousness, weakness). Treatment of mild hypoglycemia may be accomplished by consuming foods with 15–20 g of glucose (4 ounces (1/2 cup) of fruit juice or soda, 4 teaspoons of sugar, 2 tablespoons of raisins, 5 or 6 pieces of hard candy), waiting 15 minutes, and then rechecking. Glucose tablets are preferred for mild hypoglycemia, but glucose gel might be more appropriate for moderate cases. Consuming protein-rich foods is not useful to correct hypoglycemic episodes (B). Glucagon injection (A) and transportation to the emergency department (D) are reserved for severe hypoglycemia where patients are unresponsive or unable to take glucose by mouth.

62. **D.** Temperature (A), overproduction of red blood cells (polycythemia, B), and variations in hematocrit (C) have all been shown to affect meter accuracy.

164

Section 4: Answer Key

63. **D.** Patients with severe nonproliferative as well as proliferative retinopathy should avoid strenuous high-impact activities, valsalva maneuvers, and activities that jar the head (A, B, C). Low-impact aerobic exercises (D) are recommended.

64. **A.** Test once weekly at different times (A) is correct. This patient is well controlled on a stable dose of metformin; therefore, frequent self-monitored blood glucose (SMBG) testing is not necessary (C). Spot testing throughout the week at different times will help identify problems in between clinic visits. Although patients should check their blood glucose levels when symptoms of hypoglycemia occur, this should not be the only testing (D). Postprandial SMBG testing should be performed 1 to 2 hours after eating to avoid spurious results related to diet content (B).

65. **A.** Studies have shown that incorrect coding can result in errors in insulin dosing at least 10% of the time (A). Although most of the newer meters on the market are no-code or auto-code meters, a number of meters that require coding are still available for purchase (B). Newer no-code meters have been shown to be similar in accuracy to meters requiring coding by the user (C). Coding a meter calibrates the meter to the lot of strips being used. It does not determine the accuracy (D).

66. **B.** Repeat A1C today and every 3 months thereafter (B) is correct. Quarterly testing of A1C is recommended for patients who are not meeting their goals or whose therapy is changing. Not only is this patient above her A1C goal, but also her insulin regimen is constantly changing in response to metabolic demands. Quarterly A1C levels are especially important for those patients who do not have access to continuous glucose monitoring devices.

67. **C.** Single-use auto-disabling lancets that permanently retract upon puncture add an extra layer of safety in prevention of transmission of blood-borne pathogens. Removing the endcap of the lancing device between patients (A), cleaning with 70% alcohol solutions (B), and advancing pre-loaded cartridges between patients (D) are not effective precautions.

68. **B.** Renal dysfunction (B) is correct. Metformin would not be indicated for this patient due to the significance of her chronic kidney disease (CKD) as evidenced by her elevated serum creatinine (1.8 mg/dL) and albuminuria. Her ability to walk daily without chest pain or shortness of breath indicates that she does not have heart failure that would preclude metformin use (A). Patients less than 80 years old (D) and those with osteoporosis (C) are good candidates for metformin.

69. **D.** This is the correct answer due to the risk of hypoglycemia. During preconception and pregnancy, goals should be lower to prevent pregnancy-related complications (A, C). In general, the longer the life expectancy, the lower the goals as long as the person has adequate awareness of, knows how to treat, and is willing to treat hypoglycemic symptoms (B).

Review Guide for the CDE® Exam

70. **A.** Fat (A) is correct. Orlistat inhibits gastrointestinal lipases, resulting in decreased hydrolysis of dietary fat, a step necessary for absorption. Patients who consume >30% of calories as fat may experience spotting, flatus with discharge, fecal urgency, oily stool, and fecal incontinence.

71. **B.** Reduce total daily insulin dose (TDD) by ~25% (25% of 32 units = 8 units. 32 units − 8 units = 24 units); reduce the units by 50% (50% of 24 units = 12 units) and then divide by 24 hours (12 units/24 hours = 0.5).

72. **D.** TDD is divided into 450 or 500 to determine how many grams of carbohydrate are covered by 1 unit of insulin (ICR or insulin to carbohydrate ratio).

    500/32 = 15.6 units

    Alternatively, if we had the patient's weight we could have determined the insulin to carbohydrate ratio with the following formula:

    2.8 × weight (lbs)/TDD = ICR

73. **B.** The insulin sensitivity factor (ISF) or insulin correction factor (ICF) predicts how much 1 unit of insulin will lower the blood glucose of a patient. For this patient:

    Total daily insulin dose (TDD) TDD = 32 units
    Insulin correction factor = 1700/TDD (range 1600–2200) = insulin sensitivity factor.
    1700/32 = 53 or approximately 50 units

74. **A.** The Food and Drug Administration (FDA) requires performing self-monitoring of blood glucose (SMBG) to verify an interstitial glucose result from most continuous glucose monitors before making any therapy decisions. GLP-1s and metformin do not promote hypoglycemia when used as monotherapy, so additional SMBG data would not be needed (B, D). A patient managed on diet alone would not require additional SMBG after exercising, although it may be beneficial to reinforce positive behavioral changes (C).

75. **C.** Fluoxetine (C) is correct. Lorcaserin promotes weight loss by stimulating selective serotonin (5-HT2c) receptors in the hypothalamus, resulting in decreased appetite. Coadministration of selective serotonin reuptake inhibitors (SSRI) like fluoxetine may increase risk of serotonin syndrome. Statins (atorvastatin, A), biguanides (metformin, B), and angiotensin-converting enzyme (ACE) inhibitors (lisinopril, D) do not interact with lorcaserin.

76. **A.** Basal needs are evaluated fasting or preprandially. Self-monitoring of blood glucose (SMBG) performed before and 1–2 hours after a meal helps determine if meds targeted to postprandial hyperglycemia such as repaglinide need to be adjusted (B), if insulin-to-carb ratios need to adjusted (C), and the effect of the previous meal on blood glucose levels (D).

SECTION 4: ANSWER KEY

166

Section 4: Answer Key

77. **A.** Take with food or milk (A) is correct. Metformin is associated with abdominal bloating, nausea, cramping, feeling of fullness, and diarrhea—side effects that are experienced in up to 30% of users. These side effects are less with the extended release formulation, and the presence of food or milk in the stomach often attenuates these symptoms.

78. **A.** Lowering the prelunch dose of repaglinide, an insulin secretagogue, will reduce the risk of hypoglycemia. There would be no benefit in reducing the metformin (B, D). Adding snacks or increasing calories can potentially increase SW's weight or at the least hamper his efforts at weight control (C).

79. **B.** Linagliptin (B) is correct. All of the DPP-4 inhibitors may be prescribed for patients with decreased kidney function, but linagliptin does not require any dose changes due to excretion via the bile. Metformin is not recommended in patients with decreased renal function or the elderly due to increased risk of lactic acidosis (A). Although pioglitazone is eliminated through the liver and does not cause hypoglycemia, it is associated with an increased risk of osteoporotic fractures in women (C). Canagliflozin increases the risk of orthostasis, especially in the elderly, which could result in a fall (D).

80. **D.** Individuals with type 1 diabetes also are prone to Hashimoto thyroiditis, vitiligo, and celiac sprue, as well as Graves disease, autoimmune hepatitis, myasthenia gravis, and pernicious anemia.

81. **D.** Medicare Part B covers up to 100 strips every 3 months for non-insulin users after meeting the deductible, but she may get an exception if she needs more strips. For insulin users, Medicare covers up to 100 strips every month (B).

82. **D.** Glipizide (D) is correct. Although cause and effect cannot be determined, several drugs used to treat diabetes are associated with increased cancer risk: pioglitazone with increased risk of bladder cancer (A), liraglutide with increased risk of thyroid tumors (B), and sitagliptin with increased risk of pancreatic cancer (C). In each case, there is considerable uncertainty about the underlying prevalence of these cancers in the general population of patients with diabetes; therefore, the observed incidence may result from observation bias.

83. **B.** Alternate site testing can be used some of the time, but should not be used exclusively in individuals with a risk of hypoglycemia, especially when hypoglycemia is suspected or when glucose levels are changing rapidly. The educator should review which areas of the finger would cause less discomfort (A), ensure that JC is using a fine gauge lancet and changing it frequently (C), and ensure that she is using a lancing device that gives her the option of a shallow puncture depth (D).

84. **D.** Advise him that tadalafil is contraindicated with nitrates and contact his physician (D) is correct. Over half of men with diabetes report some degree of erectile dysfunction within 10 years of diagnosis. These symptoms are often an early indication of vascular damage in the coronary arteries. Agents such as sildenafil, vardenafil (B), and tadalafil are similarly effective and help restore erectile function by inhibiting breakdown of nitric oxide. Patients taking nitrates concurrently with these agents may experience

Review Guide for the CDE® Exam

severe hypotension and fatal cardiac events. Yohimbine helps patients achieve erections by increasing systemic blood pressure, which would not be a good choice in this patient with hypertension and coronary artery disease (A). Although psychosocial issues should be addressed in patients with erectile dysfunction, counseling would not be considered a substitute for drug therapy (C).

85. **B.** Omega-3 fatty acid supplements (DHA and EPA) are considered safe and beneficial for patients with diabetes and cardiovascular disease. However, there is no clear evidence of the benefit of vitamin or mineral supplementation in people with diabetes who do not have documented deficiencies, and there may be safety concerns regarding the long-term use of antioxidant supplements such as vitamins E and C and carotene (A, C, D).

86. **C.** Current recommendations include the use of glucose as the preferred treatment for the conscious individual with hypoglycemia, although any form of carbohydrate that contains glucose can be used. Consumption of 15–20 grams of carbohydrate is the recommended dosage. Fifteen minutes after treatment, if self-monitoring of blood glucose (SMBG) shows continued hypoglycemia, the treatment should be repeated. Eating until symptoms resolve frequently results in excessive hyperglycemia (A). The use of protein does not aid in the treatment of hypoglycemia (B). Glucagon injections are the recommended treatment by family members or caregivers in severe situations where the individual is unable to self-manage/self-treat (D).

87. **C.** Check her blood glucose and treat hypoglycemia if present (C) is correct. Symptoms of hypoglycemia and evolving myocardial infarctions may appear the same. Patients with symptoms related to excessive sympathetic stimulation should check their blood glucose level first, to determine the true cause. Because patients with type 2 diabetes are at high risk of coronary events, providers must first rule out cardiac causes. Eating a candy bar (A) or chewing glucose tablets (D) before checking the blood glucose will obscure the evaluation. Blindly injecting additional insulin without known blood glucose levels is never wise (B).

88. **A.** Optimal control of both glucose levels and blood pressure will slow the progression of retinopathy (A) is the correct answer. Blurry vision is due to the instability of blood glucose levels and resulting osmotic changes in the lens of the eye (B). Proliferative retinopathy, not macular edema, is characterized by neovascularization (C). Strenuous, high-impact activities and activities that involve valsalva maneuvers are contraindicated for individuals with active retinopathy (D).

89. **A.** Patients often take their premeal insulin during or after they eat a meal, resulting in hyperglycemia before the insulin has a chance to become effective. Taking lispro 10–15 minutes before eating breakfast can help prevent this problem. Adding a mid-morning snack would likely worsen the hyperglycemia (B). Increasing the basal insulin would lower his glucose throughout the day, which may not be desirable (C). Exercising in the morning may alleviate his morning hyperglycemia, but the response may not be as predictable and exercising at that time may not fit into his school schedule (D).

Section 4: Answer Key

90. **C.** Increase to 46 units (C) is correct. This patient on metformin plus glargine has a fasting blood glucose level that is significantly above his goal of <130 mg/dL as recommended by the American Diabetes Association (ADA). The treatment algorithm recommends increasing insulin doses by 10% to 15% for patients not at goal (decreasing the dose (A) would not be appropriate). Increasing the bedtime dose by only 1 unit would not likely correct the fasting hyperglycemia (B). Likewise, moving the dose to morning does not address the insufficiency of the current total daily insulin dose (D).

91. **D.** The ADA premeal target range of 80–130 mg/dL better reflects new data comparing actual average glucose levels with an A1C target of less than 7%.

92. **A.** Amlodipine (A) is correct. Data supporting the cardiovascular benefits of angiotensin-converting enzyme (ACE) inhibitors and thiazide diuretics in patients with diabetes are strong. For those patients not achieving their blood pressure goals, typically <140/90 mm Hg, addition of calcium channel blocking agents is appropriate. Peripheral vasodilators (doxazosin, B; and hydralazine, D) lower blood pressure, but lack positive cardiovascular outcomes evidence. Furosemide (C) may replace thiazide diuretics in patients with estimated glomerular filtration rates (eGFR) <30 mL/min.

93. **B.** Evidence supports encouraging individuals with diabetes to spend less time sitting (ie, watching TV, working at a computer) and add breaks when sitting longer than 90 minutes at one time. Resistance or weight training is recommended at least twice/week (A, C). Studies support the benefits for adults over the age of 18 years of performing aerobic physical activity for at least 75 minutes/week at a vigorous intensity or at least 150 minutes/week at a moderate intensity (D).

94. **A.** Both ACE inhibitors and ARBs have been shown to delay the progression of diabetic nephropathy. Low protein diets have been shown to improve albuminuria, but do not appear to have a significant effect on GFR (B). Intensive glycemic control along with improved blood pressure control delays the progression of kidney damage in patients with diabetes (C). Combination therapy with an ACE inhibitor plus an ARB worsens kidney function and should be avoided based on data from the ONTARGET study (D).

95. **C.** Rosuvastatin 20 mg (C) is correct. This patient with diabetes and a history of myocardial infarction is at very high risk and would benefit most from a high-intensity statin. Pravastatin (A), fluvastatin (B), and lovastatin (C) are all considered low intensity at the 20 mg dose.

96. **C.** Sugar alcohols are only partially absorbed, have fewer calories (B), and have less effect on blood glucose levels (A); therefore, only 1/2 the grams of sugar alcohols need to be counted (if >5 g) when basing the premeal insulin dose on the amount of carbohydrate to be consumed. There is not strong evidence to support use of sugar alcohols for weight loss or for improvement in overall glycemic control (D).

Review Guide for the CDE® Exam

97. **D.** Switch to rosuvastatin 20 mg daily (D) is correct. This patient with diabetes and a history of myocardial infarction is at very high risk and would benefit most from a high-intensity statin. Although increasing simvastatin to 80 mg daily would lower his cholesterol levels, the high dose is also associated with significantly increased risk of myositis, a problem that this patient already experienced with atorvastatin (B). Because his triglyceride levels are at goal, adding fish oil (A) or fenofibrate (C) would not be beneficial.

98. **D.** Advanced carbohydrate counting is used for intensive insulin management including individuals on multiple daily injections or pump therapy. Patients must be willing to check blood glucose numerous times a day to make informed decisions regarding insulin dosage based on blood glucose records and carbohydrate consumed. A basic approach like basic carbohydrate counting would be more appropriate for a newly diagnosed type 2 individual (A). Advanced carbohydrate counting requires a fairly high level of literacy and numeracy (C). Individuals on mixed insulin or fixed insulin regimens would not benefit from advanced carbohydrate counting since they would not adjust mealtime insulin based on their carbohydrate intake (B, C).

99. **C.** Lispro (C) is correct. Lispro, aspart, and glulisine are rapid-acting insulin products with the shortest onset, approximately 5 to 15 minutes after subcutaneous injection. The onset of regular insulin (D) is approximately 30 to 60 minutes, while intermediate-acting insulin products take 2 to 3 hours (A and B).

100. **D.** Sodium does not influence the glycemic effect of a food. Fiber (A), ripeness of fruits (B), and cooking time of starches (C) have all been studied and shown to affect glycemia.

101. **B.** Strict glycemic control has been shown to prevent the development of neuropathy in patients with type 1 diabetes. Patients with type 2 diabetes should be screened at diagnosis and then annually (A). For patients with type 1 diabetes, screening should begin 5 years after diagnosis. Electrophysiological testing is rarely needed (C). There are medications (D) available to achieve pain reduction and improve quality of life.

102. **C.** Decrease bedtime insulin glargine (C) is correct. Nocturnal hypoglycemia is a significant issue for patients and must be addressed regardless of the current A1C level (D). The basal insulin (glargine) inhibits hepatic glucose output and determines the fasting blood glucose level. Neither the breakfast (A) nor the lunchtime (B) bolus insulin doses will affect fasting glucose value.

103. **C.** The literature is mixed on the impact of high and low glycemic index/glycemic load due to the number of variables that affect the glycemic response. Research studies vary in the definitions of high, moderate, and low glycemic index or load, making it difficult to interpret study results (A). In general, fruits, sugars, and sweets have been shown to have a moderate or low glycemic effect compared with white bread or glucose (B). Research has also shown that the glycemic response to a food varies from individual to individual (D).

170

Section 4: Answer Key

104. **D.** Heart failure (D) is correct. The most serious risk related to metformin therapy is lactic acidosis. Because both metformin and lactic acid are eliminated through the kidney, disease states that decrease kidney function represent contraindications to metformin. Patients with estimated glomerular filtration rates (eGFR) greater than 30 mL/min are safe to take metformin; this patient has an eGFR of 95–102 mL/min depending on the formula employed (C). Although hypertension can worsen kidney disease, it is not a contraindication to metformin therapy (B). Severe liver dysfunction may also predispose patients to metabolic acidosis; however, the consumption reported by this patient is not problematic (A).

105. **C.** The American Diabetes Association (ADA) suggests that people with diabetes limit or avoid sugar-sweetened beverages including high-fructose corn syrup to reduce the risk for weight gain and worsening of cardiometabolic risk profile. Fructose is a monosaccharide, not a disaccharide, and part of the sucrose molecule (A). It may cause less of a rise in glucose compared with sucrose or starch (B). Consumption of excessive amounts of fructose (>12% of energy) may increase triglycerides (D).

106. **B.** Exenatide (B) is correct. GLP-1 agonists slow gastrointestinal motility and promote satiety centrally resulting in weight loss of up to 5 lbs per year. Meglitinides (nateglinide, C) and sulfonylureas (glipizide, D) promote weight gain in patients who continue to consume excess calories after starting these agents. Thiazolidinediones (TZDs) (pioglitazone, A) activate PPAR-gamma receptors that promote deposition of free fatty acids into subcutaneous adipose tissue. Deposition of free fatty acids reduces circulating plasma levels, leading to improved insulin resistance, but also results in weight gain.

107. **D.** Glucoses greater than 240 mg/dL have been shown to impair gastric emptying (A). A solid-phase gastric emptying study is the most specific way to diagnose delayed gastric emptying (C). Medical nutrition therapy (B) includes the use of multiple, small, and mostly liquid meals eaten throughout the day.

108. **B.** Resistance or strength training is used to improve muscular fitness and includes free weights, weight machines, resistance bands, isometric exercises, and calisthenics using body weight as resistance (ie, push-ups). Cycling, jogging, and sprinting are examples of aerobic exercises (A, C, D).

109. **A.** Weight loss (A) is correct. Pioglitazone is associated with multiple side effects, including bladder cancer (B), heart failure exacerbation (C), and osteoporosis and increased fracture risk (D).

110. **D.** For example, walking slowly at a lower intensity prior to a brisk walk would be an example of a proper warm-up activity. It is unclear whether stretching reduces risk of injury (A). The warm-up allows a gradual increase of the heart rate and breathing (B). Although flexibility or stretching exercises can be included as part of the warm-up, they alone are not a recommended type of warm-up activity (C).

Review Guide for the CDE® Exam

111. **D.** Add predinner (6 PM) aspart (D) is correct. This patient has fasting and predinner (6 PM) blood glucoses that are at goal, but her bedtime values are elevated. Increasing her detemir doses will result in hypoglycemia 8 to 10 hours later (A and B). Because the duration of action for metformin is so long, moving the evening dose from 6 PM to 10 PM will not affect glycemic control. The most likely cause of the elevated bedtime (10 PM) blood glucose levels is inadequate mealtime insulin.

112. **B.** Repaglinide (B) is correct. Repaglinide is a short-acting secretagogue that increases release related to meals. The other three agents primarily improve fasting blood glucose levels. Pioglitazone (A) decreases insulin resistance, metformin (C) inhibits hepatic glucose output, and glargine (D) increases circulating basal insulin levels.

113. **A.** NPH insulin 16 units at bedtime (A) is correct. Initiation of insulin for patients with type 2 diabetes should begin with basal insulin using an intermediate or long-acting product. Regular insulin may be used to cover meals or correct for glucose excursions, but would not be appropriate on a scheduled basis (B). A dose of 10 units or 0.2 units per kg is appropriate for most patients; however, a higher weight-based dose of 0.25 or 0.3 units per kg may be appropriate for obese patients.

114. **B.** Although prior recommendations stated that individuals with severe peripheral neuropathy should avoid weight-bearing activities to lower their risk of foot ulceration, recent studies show that moderate-intensity walking does not increase risk of foot ulcers and may delay the progression of peripheral neuropathy (A). Individuals with a foot injury or open sore should avoid weight-bearing exercises (C). Use of chair exercises exclusively is not necessary in all individuals with severe peripheral neuropathy (D).

115. **D.** Oral health complications of diabetes include severe periodontitis and tooth loss (A), gingivitis (B), and dental abscesses (C), but not higher rates of dental caries.

116. **C.** One unit to lower glucose to target range, plus 3.5 units to cover the carbohydrates (CHO) in the meal.

117. **B.** Increases glucagon secretion from alpha cells (B) is correct. Agents that mimic GLP-1 activity improve glycemic control through 4 actions: 1) promote satiety in the brain (A); 2) decrease glucagon secretion (B); 3) decrease gastric emptying (C); and, 4) enhance insulin secretion (D).

118. **D.** Resistance exercises such as push-ups would not be recommended due to the risk of triggering vitreous hemorrhage or retinal detachment. Swimming, stationary cycling, and walking on a treadmill would not pose significant risk (A, B, C).

119. **C.** Sitagliptin (C) is correct. This patient has New York Heart Association (NYHA) class III heart failure, which is characterized by fatigue, shortness of breath, and angina with minimal exertion. Metformin (B) and canagliflozin (A) depend on renal elimination, which may be reduced in this patient with heart failure and chronic kidney disease. Rosiglitazone may worsen symptoms of heart failure (D).

Section 4: Answer Key

120. **C.** Nuchal translucency is an ultrasonographic screening test that measures the fetal nuchal translucency thickness (skinfold area behind the nape of the neck). The test is performed at 10 to 14 weeks' gestation and is a risk predictor for chromosomal abnormalities and congenital cardiac defects. A, B, and D are all forms of fetal surveillance that access fetal well-being.

121. **A.** A 1,000-calorie deficit would likely be too aggressive for MR considering her age because it may worsen her sarcopenia, bone density, and other nutrient deficits (A). A modest reduction in calories would be more appropriate (C). Evidence supports the fact that many older adults have inadequate intakes of calcium, vitamin D, and protein (B, D).

122. **B.** Metformin (B) is correct. Insulin is considered the safest pharmacothearpy option during pregnancy; however, many patients prefer a trial with oral agents. Glyburide and metformin possess efficacy and safety data supporting their short-term use during pregnancy (B). Several other oral agents (canagliflozin, A; repaglinide, C; pioglitazone, D) lack human data supporting their use.

123. **C.** The diabetes educator should not determine the plan alone. It is important for the diabetes educator to involve the patient, the healthcare team, referring provider, and the family (as appropriate) (A, B) in deciding what will be included in the educational plan. The plan should also include specific interventions and goals (D).

124. **B.** NPH insulin (B) is correct. Exenatide and liraglutide (A) are classified in pregnancy category C and should be used during pregnancy only if the potential benefit justifies the risk. All insulin products are pregnancy category B except for glargine and glulisine, which are labeled C.

125. **C.** Asking your patient various questions about the label can provide information about her literacy level, assuming she has reading glasses available if needed. Asking your patient about her educational level or if she is able to read can cause unnecessary embarrassment and potentially elicit incorrect responses (A, B, D).

126. **D.** Methyldopa (D) is correct. Angiotensin-converting enzyme (ACE) inhibitors (lisinopril, A; fosinopril, C) and angiotensin receptor blockers (valsartan, B) are contraindicated during pregnancy because they may cause fetal harm. Antihypertensive drugs known to be effective and safe in pregnancy include methyldopa, labetalol, diltiazem, clonidine, and prazosin.

127. **C.** Reduced lung function is the unique symptom of cystic fibrosis-related diabetes (CFRD). Polyuria, polydipsia, and fatigue are symptoms of diabetes and CFRD.

128. **C.** Propranolol (C) is correct. Non-specific beta-blockers may mask sympathetic symptoms such as tachycardia associated with hypoglycemia causing patients to be unaware of low blood glucose levels.

173

Review Guide for the CDE® Exam

129. **B.** Metformin does not cause weight gain and does not promote hypoglycemia when used as monotherapy, alleviating two of BJ's problems. Glipizide XL and glimeperide are insulin secretagogues and can cause hypoglycemia and weight gain (A, C). Giving BG a mid-afternoon snack might help prevent hypoglycemia, but may sabotage her efforts at weight loss. Also, changing or adjusting medication is preferred to adding snacks to prevent hypoglycemia in overweight/obese individuals with type 2 diabetes (D).

130. **A.** Food selection to optimize glycemia should not compromise healthy eating. Avoiding major food groups such as fruits, whole grains, and dairy products can result in nutrient inadequacies and deficiencies (B). Vitamin and mineral supplements do not replace all the micronutrients and fiber present in carbohydrate foods like fruits, low-fat dairy products, and whole grains (C). The American Diabetes Association (ADA) does not recommend avoiding all foods labeled with a moderate or high glycemic index to improve glycemia (D).

131. **D.** Progestin-only contraceptives have been associated with an accelerated progression to type 2 diabetes among breastfeeding women with a history of GDM.

132. **A.** Dry hacking cough (A) is correct. Approximately 10% to 20% of patients who start on an angiotensin-converting enzyme (ACE) inhibitor experience a dry hacking cough due to accumulation of bradykinin. Although this side effect is not dangerous, it may prompt patients to switch to an antihypertensive from a different drug class. More serious side effects that would prompt immediate attention include angioedema (swelling of the face and tongue, B), hyperkalemia (high levels of potassium in the blood, C), and acute renal injury (D).

133. **D.** Specific suggestions that identify what you want them to do, how often, and how much facilitate better understanding than vague suggestions (A, B, C).

134. **C.** Fenofibrate 145 mg daily (C) is correct. Patients with triglyceride levels greater than 500 mg/dL are at high risk of pancreatitis. The first choice of drug therapy for elevated triglyceride levels is fibric acid derivatives (fenofibrate, C) or omega-3 fatty acids (fish oil). Statins (atorvastatin, A; pitavastatin, B) are considered first line to lower cardiovascular risk but have little impact on triglycerides. Ezetimibe (D) primarily lowers LDL cholesterol levels and is most useful as adjunctive therapy to statins in patients at high risk of cardiovascular events.

135. **B.** Men with diabetes tend to develop erectile dysfunction 10 to 15 years earlier than men without diabetes. As men with diabetes age, erectile dysfunction becomes even more common. As many as 75% of men and 35% of women (C) experience sexual problems related to diabetes neuropathy. Diabetes educators need to address sexual concerns because these issues may be difficult for patients to discuss (D) and this includes teens and young adults (A).

SECTION 4: ANSWER KEY

174

Section 4: Answer Key

136. **D.** Weight loss is more effective in individuals recently diagnosed who are primarily insulin resistant, with less effect among those with insulin deficiency (A, C). The Diabetes Prevention Trials showed that a weight loss of only 7–10% can help prevent diabetes (B).

137. **D.** Limit amount of dietary fiber (D) is correct. Lifestyle modifications for patients with diabetes and dyslipidemia focus on limiting cholesterol (B), saturated fat (A), and trans fat intake, while increasing viscous fiber (D), plant sterols and stanols (C), and omega-3 fatty acids.

138. **C.** Adults with uncontrolled type 2 diabetes with a BMI >35 kg/m2 may be considered for bariatric surgery, especially if the diabetes or associated conditions are difficult to control with nutrition therapy and pharmacologic therapy. Bariatric surgery is not recommended by the American Diabetes Association (ADA) for children at any age (A, D).

139. **C.** Gemfibrozil (C) is correct. Gemfibrozil inhibits glucuronidation of some lipophilic statins, resulting in elevated plasma statin levels and myositis. The risk of muscle pain is less with fenofibrate than gemfibrozil. Cholestyramine (A), ezetimibe (B), and omega-3 fatty acids or fish oil (D) do not inhibit statin metabolism or increase the risk of myositis.

140. **C.** Higher remission rates of diabetes are associated with a shorter duration of type 2 diabetes with younger age, lower A1C, higher serum insulin levels, and nonuse of insulin (B and D). Diabetes remission rates are also higher with procedures that bypass portions of the small intestine than with those that only restrict the stomach. Body mass index (BMI) is not a strong predictor of remission (A).

141. **B.** Activity focus should be on enjoyable playtime activity rather than structured exercise bouts including school sports, recreational leagues, and active family outings (A, C, D).

142. **D.** Hypoglycemia (D) is correct. Niacin causes prostaglandin-mediated vasodilation that patients report as "hot flashes" or flushing (A). At therapeutic doses, niacin may increase uric acid levels (C) and elevate liver transaminase levels (B).

143. **C.** The Academy of Nutrition and Dietetics (AND) Evidence-Based Nutrition Practice Guidelines for Diabetes recommend that persons with either type 1 or type 2 diabetes who adjust their mealtime insulin or who are on insulin pump therapy should adjust their insulin doses to match carbohydrate intake (insulin-to-carbohydrate ratio).

144. **B.** Take aspirin 325 mg about 30 minutes before niacin (B) is correct. Niacin causes prostaglandin-mediated vasodilation that patients report as "hot flashes" or flushing. Aspirin inhibits prostaglandin synthesis and abates the flushing effect. Patients should also be advised to take niacin on a full stomach to delay dose absorption over a longer period of time. Actions that promote peripheral vasodilation, such as hot showers (C) or beverages (D), will worsen flushing symptoms. Tachyphylaxis develops to the niacin flush over time; however, discontinuing niacin will cause the flush to return with the following doses (A).

175

Review Guide for the CDE® Exam

145. **A.** In addition, the recommendations include initiation of testing at age 10 or at onset of puberty. The recommended A1C testing frequency is every 3 years.

146. **B.** Fish oil (B) is correct. Omega-3 fatty acids or fish oil appears to act as a naturally occurring ligand for PPAR-alpha, which promotes lipoprotein lipase activity and reduces triglyceride levels. Garlic (A) modestly lowers total cholesterol, but does not affect triglyceride levels. Ezetimibe (C) and plant sterols (D) primarily lower LDL cholesterol.

147. **D.** Four risk factors (D) is correct. Traditional risk factors for cardiovascular disease are age, family history, smoking, hypertension, and serum HDL cholesterol. This patient is a man over 45 years old with a family history of cardiovascular disease, hypertension, and low HDL cholesterol (<40 mg/dL).

148. **D.** Lack of motivation is a barrier in all socioeconomic groups. The cost of gym membership or gym equipment may affect exercise opportunities in low socioeconomic groups (A). Inability to walk in unsafe neighborhoods and proximity or access to gyms due to location or transportation issues can impact exercise opportunities (B, C).

149. **B.** Abdominal aortic aneurysm (B) is correct. Patients with peripheral arterial disease, history of abdominal aortic aneurysm, metabolic syndrome, or Framingham 10-year risk score (D) of >20% are considered to have the same atherosclerotic cardiovascular disease (ASCVD) risk as patients with established coronary artery disease (CAD). Other biomarkers of cardiovascular disease (hs-CRP, C; ankle brachial index <0.9, A) may help modify goals of therapy, but do not establish absolute risk by themselves.

150. **C.** Metformin has a long-standing evidence base for efficacy and safety, is inexpensive, and may reduce risk of cardiovascular events. According to ADA guidelines, metformin is the preferred initial pharmacologic agent for type 2 diabetes.

151. **B.** Women with gestational diabetes who are overweight or obese can reduce their risk of type 2 diabetes with postpartum weight loss. The risk of offspring with cystic fibrosis or heart defects is not increased in women with gestational diabetes (A, D). Gestational diabetes is not known to increase the risk of obesity, but obesity can increase the risk of gestational diabetes (C).

152. **A.** Fish that contain high levels of methyl-mercury, such as swordfish, shark, and tilefish, should be avoided during pregnancy. Mercury crosses the placenta and can damage the fetal nervous system. Studies do not support the need for all organic foods during pregnancy (B). Raw fruits and vegetables, if washed thoroughly, do not pose a threat to the fetus (C). Salmon is considered one of the fish lower in mercury levels (D).

153. **D.** Colesevelam (D) is correct. Selection of drug therapy during pregnancy must consider both the mother and the developing fetus. Bile acid sequestrants reduce cholesterol by binding biliary cholesterol in the gastrointestinal tract. These agents are not systemically absorbed and would be better choices than other options that may pass across the placenta. Rosuvastatin, gemfibrozil, and niacin are contraindicated during pregnancy (A, B, C).

SECTION 4: ANSWER KEY

176

Section 4: Answer Key

154. **B.** Since MS is normally fairly inactive, she would be advised to engage in activities such as walking for 30 minutes most days of the week (A). If she regularly engaged in vigorous activity prior to the pregnancy, she would be advised to continue the activity provided she and the baby remained healthy and discussed with her healthcare provider adjustments in activity over time (C). MS would not be restricted to flexibility exercises and upper body exercises unless she had complications (D).

155. **A.** These foods all contain gluten, which damages the intestinal epithelium, causing abdominal pain, diarrhea, malabsorption, and failure to thrive. The sodium content of a food does not affect children with celiac disease (B). Rice and corn do not contain gluten (C, D).

156. **B.** Because of the long history of type 1 diabetes and the classic symptoms she describes, it appears that she is experiencing gastroparesis, a form of autonomic neuropathy. IBS, GERD, or a virus would not explain her episodes of hypoglycemia following a meal (A, C, D).

157. **A.** Although physical activity can acutely increase urinary protein excretion (D), there is no evidence that vigorous excessive increases the rate of progression of diabetic kidney disease. In the presence of proliferative diabetic retinopathy, vigorous aerobic or resistance exercise is contraindicated because of the risk of triggering vitreous hemorrhage or retinal detachment (A). Peripheral neuropathy (C) with the associated decrease in sensation carries an increased risk of injury; however, moderate-intensity walking may not increase the risk of foot ulcer formation. Diabetic gastroparesis (B) is unaffected by activity level.

158. **A.** Fish oil (A) is correct. This patient currently takes a high-intensity statin but remains above his goal of non-HDL cholesterol of less than 100 mg/dL. His primary lipoprotein abnormality is a triglyceride greater than 500 mg/dL, which increases not only his cardiovascular risk but also his risk for pancreatitis. Both fluvastatin (B) and simvastatin (C) are less effective than rosuvastatin and do not offer additional triglyceride reduction. Adding colesevelam (D) would help lower the LDL cholesterol, but might also cause the triglyceride level to rise, increasing the risk of pancreatitis.

159. **B.** He is willing to make some of the recommended changes within the next 6 months and is aware of the benefits and the costs of change.

160. **B.** Since the woman is experiencing some hypoglycemia in the middle of the night and early morning, she should have her bedtime insulin reduced. Although some of her fasting blood sugar (FBS) are elevated, this appears to likely be a rebound from unrecognized hypoglycemia.

161. **D.** Metformin (D) is correct. This patient has an A1C value that is 1.8% away from her goal. Biguanides (metformin, D) and sulfonylureas lower A1C by approximately 1% to 2%, whereas GLP-1 agonists (exenatide, A), DPP-4 inhibitors (saxagliptin, B), and alphaglucosidase inhibitors (acarbose, C) lower A1C by 0.5% to 1%.

177

Review Guide for the CDE® Exam

162. **D.** Nateglinide is an insulin secretagogue and is associated with weight gain. Exenatide, a GLP-1 agonist, can result in weight loss (A), and metformin and acarbose inhibitors are considered weight neutral (B, C).

163. **D.** Insulin pump therapy is more effective than multiple daily injections because of the ability to vary basal insulin delivery (D).

164. **C.** Baked products and canned biscuits are frequently made with artificial trans fats. Check the Nutrition Facts label for trans fats and also the ingredient label for hydrogenated or partially hydrogenated oils. Liquid margarines, liquid soybean oil, and avocados do not contain artificial trans fats (A, B, D).

165. **B.** Sitagliptin (B) is correct. Exogenous insulin (D) and insulin secretagogues (glyburide, A; repaglinide, C) are associated with increased likelihood of hypoglycemia. Inhibitors of the DPP-4 enzyme improve glycemic control by stimulating glucose-dependent insulin release from the pancreas.

166. **D.** A vegan eating plan does not include fish, poultry, meat, dairy products, or eggs (A, B, C) or products made with them.

167. **C.** Secondary infection of tooth (C) is correct. During times of acute illness, glucose levels are elevated. In this patient, the A1C level is at goal, suggesting that the current diabetes regimen is appropriate. Patients taking sulfonylureas often experience secondary failure (B) characterized by a slow progressive rise in blood glucose levels that also affect A1C. Similarly, progression of diabetes is a slow process that occurs over time as beta-cell capacity to produce insulin declines (D). Although hypothyroidism may decrease insulin production, hyperthyroid states tend to cause low blood glucose levels due to increased metabolic rate (A).

168. **B.** Whole grains contain the entire grain kernel—the bran, germ, and endosperm. Refined grains are processed to remove the bran and germ along with many of the nutrients. Long-grain white rice and jasmin rice are refined grains (A, C). Honey wheat flour and white wheat flour have been processed and are therefore not considered whole grain flour unless they are preceded by the term "whole" (C, D). Flour tortillas are made with refined flour (C).

169. **B.** Canagliflozin (B) is correct. The SGLT-2 inhibitors lower blood glucose by blocking glucose reabsorption in the kidneys. Loss of glucose in the urine may promote weight loss as well as improved glycemic control. Sitagliptin (A) and the other DPP-4 inhibitors do not cause hypoglycemia but are considered weight neutral. Both long-acting glargine (C) and rapid acting glulisine insulin (D) are likely to cause hypoglycemia in patients actively attempting to lose weight.

170. **C.** Add nateglinide (C) is correct. The maximum effective dose of metformin is 2 grams per day (A). The primary reason why this patient's A1C remains above 7% is that he

Section 4: Answer Key

has insufficient insulin production in response to his large evening meal. Adding basal insulin (glargine, B) or a long-acting sulfonylurea (glyburide, D) would likely cause hypoglycemia during the day. A short-acting secretagogue would provide this patient with the most flexibility around his irregular meal schedule and avoid hypoglycemia.

171. **B.** The prelunch glucose levels are elevated and it is the prebreakfast Lispro that has the strongest action during this period.

172. **D.** The recommendation is that individuals test every 2–4 hours while symptomatic and blood glucose levels are elevated. Insulin should not be stopped or held in individuals with type 1 diabetes, as they are insulinopenic and could quickly develop diabetic ketoacidosis (DKA) (B). Eight ounces of fluid per hour is recommended to prevent dehydration (C). Carbohydrates and insulin are needed to reverse ketosis (A).

173. **C.** This individual is ready to change in the near future and is taking steps to begin making a change.

174. **B.** Thiazolidinediones cause fluid retention and edema, especially when used in combination with insulin. Patients taking TZDs have a twofold increase in the risk of heart failure. Dose-related weight gain occurs with TZDs and is thought to be related to a combination of fluid retention and subcutaneous fat accumulation.

175. **A.** This test measures a glucose-like sugar named 1,5-AG, which is found in most foods. The test assesses the amount of time over a 2-week period that glucose exceeds the renal threshold. Whenever the glucose is over 180 mg/dL the body loses 1,5-AG. The more the glucose spikes, the lower the result. Its validity is limited in patients with advanced kidney and liver disease as well as during pregnancy.

176. **D.** The Early Treatment Diabetic Retinopathy Study (ETDRS) found that aspirin had no significant effect on retinopathy.

177. **C.** Colesevelam is classified in pregnancy Category B, no evidence of risk in humans, whereas other bile acid resins (cholestyramine and colestipol) are Category C. Fenofibrate is also in pregnancy Category C (A). Atorvastatin, like all statins, is classified in pregnancy Category X and should not be used during pregnancy (B). Evolocumab is a PCSK-9 inhibitor that has not been used in pregnancy; however, IgG antibodies cross the placenta and fetal exposure to evolocumab would be expected especially in the second and third trimesters (D).

178. **A.** According to the American Diabetes Association (ADA) Practice Guidelines, insulin therapy should be initiated for the treatment of persistent hyperglycemia starting at a threshold of no greater than 180 mg/dL and the maintained in a range of 140 to 180 mg/dL. Trials in critically ill persons have failed to show a significant improvement in mortality with intensive glycemic control, but have demonstrated an increased risk of severe hypoglycemia.

Review Guide for the CDE® Exam

179. **D.** Weight loss, not weight gain, increases the risk of hypoglycemia. Risk of hypoglycemia is increased when an individual has not eaten for several hours (A), when an individual takes medications that enhance insulin secretion, and/or during periods of significantly increased physical activity (C). Alcohol consumption, without food intake, may also result in hypoglycemia (B).

180. **D.** Individuals with diabetes should be screened, advised, and assessed for readiness to quit smoking at every diabetes care visit.

181. **D.** Large trials in type 2 diabetes have demonstrated improvements in microvascular disease among individuals with tight glycemic control, but not an improvement in cardiovascular outcomes (C). Strict glycemic control is associated with a decrease in triglycerides (B) but has also been associated with weight gain (A).

182. **C.** Insulin resistance is lowest during the first trimester and increases throughout gestation, leading to increased insulin requirements. Insulin requirements drop dramatically following delivery.

183. **B.** For patients who may become hypoglycemic and are unable to mount a counter-regulatory response, the use of smaller boluses is indicated to reduce the possibility of hypoglycemia.

184. **D.** Glipizide, metformin, and acarbose, as well as glyburide, are all considered compatible with breastfeeding.

185. **D.** Diabetes-related distress is particularly common, with prevalence rates of 18% to 35% and an 18-month incidence of 38% to 48%. It has a greater impact on behavioral and metabolic outcomes than does depression. Diabetes-related distress is responsive to interventions, including DSMES and focused attention.

186. **D.** Unopened and opened vials of insulin may be stored at room temperature for 1 month (B). Regardless of whether insulin is opened or unopened it should not be used past the expiration date (C).

187. **D.** Controlled diabetes with recent physiologic stress is correct. With prolonged hyperglycemia his A1C upon admission would have been increased. As his A1C is at goal, it is unlikely due to a recent improvement (B) or insulin dose increase that would have lowered his point-of-care glucose values (C).

188. **C.** Having a CDE on staff is not a requirement although it is an advantage (A). Accreditation or recognition is required to receive Medicare reimbursement; however, it doesn't guarantee reimbursement (B). Medicare has agreed to cover diabetes education up to 10 hours in the first year, but this should not determine the program's length (D).

189. **D.** For this category of medication, category X, there is positive evidence of fetal abnormalities or risk. Category A medications have been well studied and have not shown an increased risk of abnormalities (A). Category B animal studies may have shown an adverse effect, but controlled studies in humans have found no effect (A). Category C

180

Section 4: Answer Key

animal studies may or may not have shown an effect in animals, but there are no well-controlled studies in humans (B). Category D indicates that there is evidence in human studies, indicating an increased risk to the fetus (C).

190. **D.** Bedtime intermediate-acting insulin has been shown to reduce nocturnal hypoglycemia and allow for better glucose control in the morning. Reducing his NPH before dinner (A, B) would reduce the risk of nocturnal hypoglycemia but would increase the likelihood of higher fasting glucose levels. Increasing the bedtime snack (C) would have the same effect and would not be desirable since it would increase his caloric intake while he is trying to lose weight.

191. **A.** Although glucose tolerance declines with age, the diagnostic criteria remain the same for the elderly as for the young. Older adults rarely present with the typical symptoms of hyperglycemia (C). Physiologic changes associated with aging may diminish thirst and increase dehydration. Glycosuria at the usual levels may not be seen because of the advance in renal threshold associated with aging. Slowed counter-regulation of hormones, erratic food intake, and slowed intestinal absorption place the older adult at higher risk of hypoglycemia (B). Disabilities may be directly linked to eye disease, stroke, cardiovascular disease, neuropathies, and peripheral vascular disease (D).

192. **B.** The key to successful goal setting is effective questioning around the patient's desire to make a change, the ability to make a change, the reasons for making a change, and the need to make a change.

193. **D.** Problem solving is best used when there are a variety of options or courses of action from which to choose. Direct instruction is recommended for problems that are well defined, straightforward, and/or require the professional or clinical expertise of the educator (A and B) and problems that have a known, specific course of action, such as C.

194. **A.** Even mild elevations in A1C have been associated with increased fetal morbidity.

195. **C.** Optimizing blood glucose, blood pressure, and lipid control have all been shown to slow progression and are particularly effective when initiated early. The other statements (A, B, and D) are correct.

196. **C.** Studies have shown that DSMES improves hemoglobin A1C (A1C) by as much as 1% in people with type 2 diabetes.

197. **B.** 80% of (5 units/hour × 24) = 96 units.

198. **B.** Basal dose is 50% of the total daily insulin dose. 96 units × 50% = 48 units.

199. **D.** The bolus total dose is the other 50% divided among the 3 meals. 48 units/3 meals = 16 units.

200. **A.** Subcutaneous insulin should be given before the drip is discontinued in order to allow an overlap that takes into consideration the onset of action. The first dose of basal insulin should be given 2 hours before the insulin infusion is discontinued.